QUACKS

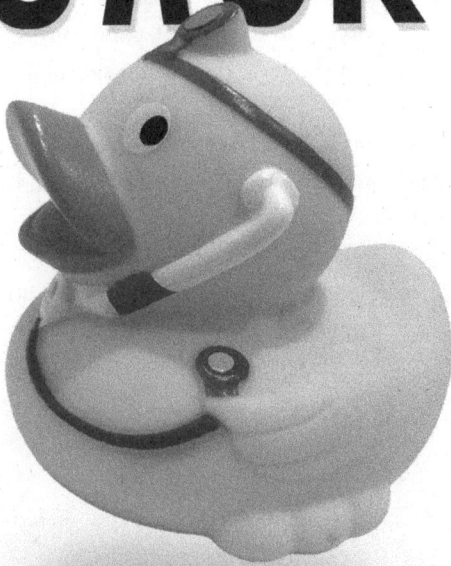

DR AHMED HANDY

CRANTHORPE
— MILLNER —
PUBLISHERS

First published by Cranthorpe Millner Publishers (2025)

ISBN 978-1-80378-286-7 (Paperback)

www.cranthorpemillner.com

Cranthorpe Millner Publishers

Printed and bound by CPI Group (UK) Ltd
Croydon, CR0 4YY

MIX
Paper | Supporting
responsible forestry
FSC
www.fsc.org
FSC® C013604

To the two incredible, defining women in my life:
my late mother, to whom I owe so much of who I am, and so
many of the opportunities I've been blessed with in life; and
my wife, without whose unwavering love and support I would
undoubtedly be a lesser man.

And to my son: your smile and warmth brighten every room,
and you've made my heart fuller than I ever thought possible.

PREFACE

Hello, my name is Dr Ahmed Handy, and I'm a General Practitioner (GP). At the risk of us getting off on the wrong foot, I feel obligated to point out that precisely fifty percent of that opening statement is a lie.

Yes, I really am a GP (currently working in the Midlands), but my name isn't really Ahmed. Why this particular pen name? Well, as the son of two Arabs, my real first name was inspired by the surname of a well-known Arabic writer called Ahmed. And Handy is a play on my late mother's maiden name.

Why have a pen name at all? The simple fact is that given that I do currently work as a GP, I would hate for the very existence of this book to in any way detract from my current job – one which I love, and feel grateful for each and every day (well, more or less). To be able to realise my childhood ambition of helping to make sick people better is an honour and a privilege, as is working for the great and enduring institution that is the NHS.

Having come across this book, you may well be thinking: "Oh God – not *another* junior doctor memoir. Jesus, have they all just become writers now, or do any of them actually still, you know, practise medicine?" And in truth, I wouldn't even blame you for thinking that. What I'd like to think makes this particular book stand apart, however, is that – unlike most other junior doctor memoirs – this one is much less focused on patients (indeed, you'll probably find less than half a dozen patient anecdotes in the ensuing chapters), or even its author, and much more focused on the doctors themselves.

You will, I'm sure, be familiar with the expression, 'You don't have to be crazy to work here – but it helps'. Well, even as a medical student, it didn't take me long at all to realise that when you're working in medicine, that's not just a truism, it's practically a prescription. Ultimately, I think we all must be a little bit crazy to stay in the (inarguably challenging) world of medicine month after month, year after year. Indeed, it's precisely that ability to embrace the absurd, and the inherently strange aspects of what we do day in day out that probably keeps many of us from letting the stresses of the job get to us, and ultimately falling apart at the seams.

It also didn't take me very long to realise that some doctors definitely embrace that madness perhaps a little *too* much – hence the title of this book, *Quacks*. The title is not, I hasten to add, meant to be taken literally; I am not at all suggesting that any of the doctors I worked with during my time as a junior doctor were frauds or charlatans (though some of their behaviours and practices most definitely did make me raise a Roger Moore-esque eyebrow on more than one occasion). Furthermore, when you live and work in certain parts of the Midlands, you very quickly get used to being referred to as 'duck' (whether or not you are indeed a waterfowl bird) – a fact that certainly stuck in my mind when considering what to call this memoir.

Ultimately, I hope you'll all take this book for what it

is meant to be: an irreverent, humorous (hopefully) and occasionally (but not too frequently) serious look at the life of a junior doctor, predominantly viewed through the prism of the very real (and often eccentric) characters I worked with along the way. Together with my own, all the names in this book (plus, consequently, the name of one particular song!) have been changed in order to protect the identities of the individuals concerned (as well as possibly protecting me from a leg breaking or two, should I ever run into some of them again). But the stories contained herein are otherwise most definitely one hundred percent real.

This book specifically covers my time working as a junior doctor in hospital, which spanned a total of just under four years. I have omitted the time I spent as a junior doctor working in the community (in both Psychiatry, and later as a trainee in General Practice), as well as in Accident & Emergency (A&E) – predominantly as I have far fewer noteworthy stories about the people I worked with during those particular clinical attachments (aka rotations). I also use the term 'junior doctor' fairly loosely in this memoir. Technically speaking, 'junior doctor' refers to pretty much any qualified doctor who is below GP or consultant level. However, for the sake of clarity, I have instead used it in the chapters that follow to refer to any doctor less qualified than a registrar. Registrars are the immediate juniors to the consultants, and I worked with (and have stories about) many of them over the years. Where possible, I have attempted to explain and/or give context to terms and concepts that are relevant to the training one undergoes as a junior doctor, though I have been deliberate in not making doing so an overly cumbersome part of this book.

Finally, as well as the people I refer to in this book's dedication, I would also like to give special mention to two other individuals. Firstly, doctor and author Dr Joanna Cannon. We worked together briefly when I did a four-month rotation in community Psychiatry, and I was struck by her warm, good-hearted nature, as well as her unfailing compassion towards the patients on the ward. In quieter moments, she would also sometimes tell me about her passion for writing, and thus I was delighted when I learned that she had released her very first book, just a few short years later. Her success certainly served as an inspiration to me when deciding to write this memoir. Secondly, my much missed friend (and fellow theatre enthusiast) Ben Dowell. Ben was sadly diagnosed with cancer in 2018, which he battled bravely for an unprecedented four years. During that incredibly difficult time, he managed to self-publish two books detailing his fascinating near thirty year career as a film projectionist and engineer, a remarkable and humbling achievement. He was one of the kindest, gentlest and most engaging people I've ever met, and I am hugely grateful to have known him.

I hope you enjoy this book – but even if you don't, thanks for reading.

PART I

CARDIOLOGY

PART 1

CARDIOLOGY

ARAB IN THE HEADLIGHTS

Thanks to the influence of our American cousins, most people are now familiar with Black Friday, the day that follows Thanksgiving (and notable mainly for the frenzied shopping sales that the day heralds). What you may not be familiar with, however, is Black *Wednesday*.

In the medical and surgical world, Black Wednesday is the first Wednesday in August. It is so-called because it is the day that eager-eyed junior doctors, fresh from medical school, start work on the hospital wards for the very first time. Unhelpfully, it is also the day when many of the more experienced ward doctors swap departments, leaving only the consultants (and a handful of other retained staff) to shoulder the responsibility of ensuring that the ward continues to run smoothly – and of showing the (mostly terrified) new junior doctors the ropes. Black Wednesday has attracted an increasing amount of media attention in recent years, with members of the public jokingly being warned not to fall ill at the start of August. Such 'warnings' are sadly not without merit. A 2013 article in *The Telegraph* reported that heart attack and stroke patients are eight percent more likely to die on Black Wednesday than they are on the preceding Wednesday.

For junior doctors, Black Wednesday inevitably feels very much like a trial by fire. And the next person to take that dreaded leap into the world of hospital medicine was me.

Five years, nine months and eleven days: that's the exact amount of time that passed between my very first day at medical school and the day I graduated as a doctor. I believed then, as I still do, that medicine is an incredibly rewarding and noble career path. However, it is not one to be undertaken lightly. It takes years of study, hard work and perseverance, not to mention a fair amount of blood, sweat and tears (in some cases, quite literally). What really took me by surprise though was just how much all that accumulated knowledge – and confidence – seemed to vanish in an instant the moment I set foot on the Cardiology ward as a qualified doctor on Black Wednesday, over a decade ago.

To make matters worse, I was the only first year junior doctor (termed a Foundation Year 1, or FY1 doctor) who would be working in Cardiology over the next four months. Although I was far from the only junior doctor on the ward, in many ways I still felt very much like I was by myself. It's at times like that you really do value having a support network of experienced senior colleagues around you. Indeed, my main hope going into that very first job was that I would have a supportive, level-headed boss to help guide me through the troubled waters I was venturing into until I felt ready to set sail alone.

Sadly, I was fresh out of luck.

JOHN WAYNE, M.D.

The consultant I was attached to, Dr Singh, was a fascinating individual in many ways – from the way he looked, to the way he walked, to the frankly bewildering things that came out of his mouth.

Despite being in his early sixties, he was a man who was clearly determined not to let the ageing process catch up with him. He had typical male pattern baldness, with greying black hair and a similarly-coloured thick bristly moustache. However, what I found most intriguing was that as the months passed, his hair became steadily blacker – an obvious dye job, made all the more noticeable by his inexplicable decision not to dye his moustache as well. Over time, his hair became the kind of unnatural jet black colour you only ever find in shoe polish. It was an odd sight to behold, especially given the stark visual contrast with his stubbornly greying moustache.

And then there was the way he walked; all distinctive wide hips and halting gait. It was a walk I have otherwise only ever seen cowboys do in old black and white westerns. Indeed, I was not the only person to notice it, and his inimitable walk soon earned Dr Singh the nickname John Wayne.

Perhaps what was most remarkable about Dr Singh was his incredible ability to appear like he was listening to you, whilst failing to take in a single word you said. One of the best examples of this came during a ward round I did with Dr Singh one Monday afternoon, just a few short weeks into my rotation.

For those of you unfamiliar with the term (and it's one you'll see often in this book), a ward round refers to when the medical or surgical team (usually led by one of the senior doctors) circumnavigates the ward(s), and sees/reviews all the patients under their care. During a ward round, the junior doctors (who see the patients every day, thereby making them largely responsible for ongoing continuity of care) are typically expected to grab each set of individual case notes as they go from bed to bed, and then 'present' each patient in turn to the doctor leading the round.

About halfway through this particular ward round, I retrieved the notes for a patient I had come to know reasonably well over the preceding few days, John Smith. I began, "Dr Singh, the next patient is John Smith. He was admitted via ambulance three days ago following an NSTEMI [a type of heart attack]. He's in bed fourteen."

Dr Singh then immediately proceeded to walk towards bed fourteen in which Mr Smith was sat upright, watching TV. Upon making eye contact with the patient, Dr Singh started waving towards him, before cheerily calling out, "Hi, Michael!"

To be honest, I'm not entirely certain who looked more befuddled in that particular moment – John Smith, or me.

I pulled the curtains around the bed as Dr Singh began inspecting Mr Smith's observation chart. It was then that Dr Singh suddenly noticed the white board behind the patient's bed. Upon it, in large black letters, was written: JOHN

SMITH.

Appearing puzzled for a moment, Dr Singh then turned to me before casually remarking, "Look at that, Ahmed – they've written the wrong name up on the board."

I was at a loss for words.

Worse was an incident that I (perhaps mercifully) was not personally witness to, but was recounted to me by a junior doctor colleague, Sarah. Sarah was already well aware of Dr Singh's seeming inability to accurately retain information, given that he repeatedly called her "Sandy" for the better part of three months.

Sarah had been on call overnight, and was presenting all the patients who had been admitted over the preceding twelve hours to Dr Singh, who happened to be the on call consultant that day.

"This next patient, Albert White, is a seventy-two-year-old gentleman who was admitted with a seven-day history of worsening shortness of breath and chest pains. He has a known diagnosis of heart failure, and we've been managing his symptoms overnight with high doses of diuretics [water tablets]." Sarah then paused, adding with deliberate emphasis, "I should also make you aware, Dr Singh, that this patient is registered blind." It was a point she emphasised precisely in the (ultimately vain) hope of avoiding what was – with excruciating inevitability – about to come next.

"Okay, Sandy," Dr Singh replied, "let's go see him."

Sarah and Dr Singh pulled back the curtains surrounding the cubicle where the patient lay in bed, wearing thick dark sunglasses.

"Hello, sir. I am Dr Singh, the consultant on call. Can you

please tell me a bit about what's brought you into hospital?"

As Mr White began recounting his story, Dr Singh immediately began checking his medication chart, presumably only half-listening to what Mr White was saying. When he'd finally finished with the chart, he looked up at the patient and suddenly appeared to notice his sunglasses for the first time. Interrupting Mr White mid-sentence, Dr Singh suddenly interjected. "Oh, can you please take off those sunglasses, sir? You obviously don't need them inside."

Perhaps my favourite story about Dr Singh though, relates to another ward round. On this occasion, he and I were joined by Phil, another junior doctor. The final patient on the round was Eric Carter, a fifty-four-year-old gentleman who had been admitted five days earlier following a heart attack; the ward manager had already flagged him to us as someone who was potentially fit for discharge home that day.

Now, as part of the medical management for patients who have suffered a heart attack, we are meant to give them general health and lifestyle advice, with a view to hopefully reducing their risk of suffering from further heart problems in future. This would typically involve us discussing so-called 'modifiable' risk factors, such as smoking, weight, diet and exercise.

Once he had established that the patient was indeed fit to be discharged home, Dr Singh paused, before giving Mr Carter a slightly disapproving look. This, presumably, was the moment when Dr Singh was going to discuss ways in which the patient could improve his lifestyle. My sense of anticipation peaked, whilst simultaneously feeling my heart in my throat.

"Okay, Mr Carter, we'll get your paperwork sorted, and

then you'll be free to go home. But if you don't want to end up back in here again in the future, just remember: don't do silly things." And with that, Dr Singh abruptly walked off, thus (apparently) ending the ward round.

As Phil and I returned to the doctors' office – both barely able to contain ourselves – I looked down to see what Phil was writing in Mr Carter's notes. Whatever it was, it was bound to be good. Sure enough, I wasn't disappointed. Towards the bottom of his entry, Phil had written the following:

Dr Singh has discussed lifestyle factors and secondary health preventative measures with the patient.

Bursting out laughing, I exclaimed, "You got *that* from 'don't do silly things'?!"

With a knowing smile, Phil replied, "Well, what would you prefer I put – the truth?"

The man had a point.

To cap it all off, around three months into my four-month rotation, Dr Singh left the department, with little notice or fanfare. As to why, I was never quite sure. The rumour mill suggested that Dr Singh had only been hired by the department on a locum (temporary) contract, and had subsequently found a job elsewhere. As befitting his cowboy moniker, I like to picture the man who was my very first boss riding off into the sunset on the back of some magnificent steed, dripping a trail of fresh black shoe polish in his wake. And with that, he was gone. To be frank, I can't say I was all that sad.

In an ironic twist of fate, about a fortnight before my rotation was due to end, another consultant – Dr Adams – was brought in to replace Dr Singh. He was friendly and supportive, and always happy to lend a helping hand. He was, in fact, quite possibly one of the nicest men in the world.

Do you remember the darts gameshow *Bullseye*? Host Jim Bowen used to do this peculiar thing where he would invite losing contestants to 'come and have a look at what you could have won', before his assistant would wheel out the Star Prize (usually a speedboat) from behind a screen, all to the sound of a sad, downbeat version of the gameshow's theme music.

It was during a ward round with Dr Adams – days away from the end of my rotation – that it suddenly dawned on me: he was what *I* could've won – my own personal speedboat. Instead, for months on end I'd been forced to make do with a badly polished, slowly sinking rowboat. Cue the sad music.

LOCK UP YOUR NURSES

Within the Cardiology department, the doctors were all divided into colour-coded teams, with each team typically consisting of a junior doctor, a registrar and a consultant. Myself and Dr Singh (and latterly Dr Adams, albeit briefly) made up the green team. Much to my chagrin, there was no registrar assigned to the green team whilst I was there – a less than ideal situation when you've never done a hospital job before, and your only other form of direct senior support is Dr Don't-Do-Silly-Things.

Each team was also expected to provide cross-cover for either one or two additional teams, in case of staff absences, or to help lighten the burden if (for a variety of reasons) one particular consultant ended up with a disproportionately large number of patients under their care compared to their colleagues.

The green team was nominally aligned with both the yellow team (whose junior doctor was the aforementioned Phil) and the blue team (whose junior, confusingly, was called Will). The fact that Phil and Will often ended up being referred to by the other's name was not exactly a surprise, especially given that they were both Caucasian men in their late twenties. What did surprise me, however, was that *I* would often be called either Phil or Will by various nurses on the ward. Each time I was, I couldn't help but think to myself, "For God's sake, just *look* at me. I mean – out of Phil, Will and Ahmed, with my complexion, which one am *I* likely to be?" Often, the nurses would cycle through all three names in quick-fire succession until they arrived at mine, to the point that I was frequently (and absentmindedly) referred to as 'Phil-Will-Ahmed'.

The consultant in charge of the yellow team (and thus someone with whom I ended up working quite closely during my Cardiology rotation) – was Dr Jackman, a well-built, handsome Kiwi in his late forties. Dr Jackman was also my very first so-called clinical supervisor; that meant, whilst he may not have been the consultant for my 'team', he was responsible for monitoring my progress over the course of my four-month attachment (and, ultimately, for signing me off as competent for progression at the end of it).

I think that most people will agree that when you start a new job, your primary goal – at least, in the beginning – is simple: don't screw it up. Though I had already spent a fair amount of time on hospital wards as a medical student, this was always going to be different. Ultimately, what you did on the wards as a medical student was largely inconsequential. You were principally there to learn, and so had no true responsibility resting on your shoulders. If you simply didn't turn up one day, then you'd often be lucky if someone even noticed, let alone it causing some kind of disruption to patient care. For most medical students, your main priority when in hospitals is picking up tips on how to pass those all-important final exams; learning the ropes as regards the more practical aspects of the junior doctor role that you would soon be taking on, a distant second. Being a fully qualified doctor was different: what you did actually mattered, and – though you were still generally well-supported – it very much felt like the training wheels were off. To say that those initial weeks and months on the job were a steep learning curve would be a massive understatement.

In some hospitals, there is a mandatory 'shadowing' period for incoming junior doctors, during which they are required to be present on the wards during the weeks preceding the official start of their job, in order to shadow the outgoing junior doctors whom they will soon be replacing. In the case of my particular hospital, however, there was no such requirement. We were only obligated to come in for a full-day hospital induction on a Tuesday, with Black Wednesday being the very next day.

Given my apprehension about going out into the big wide medical world, I decided therefore that it might be a good idea to take a modicum of initiative, and turn up on the wards a day early, on the Monday. I realised that it was debateable as to how much I could really pick up in just the one, eight-hour shift, but I reasoned that it was surely better than nothing. And so it was that I turned up, unannounced, on the ward bright and early on that first Monday in August, hungry to learn, and, crucially, eager to impress.

I genuinely don't envy the more senior doctors who work on hospital wards, for the simple reason that the onus is for ever on them to be 'keepers of the flame'. Unlike junior doctors, they don't have the (debateable) luxury of simply being able to move to another department after four (sometimes six) months; it's their job to ensure that the ward (and, most importantly, patient care) continues to run as smoothly as possible, despite the semi-frequent changes in medical staff.

The consultants in particular will have seen dozens (maybe even hundreds) of junior doctors come and go over the years. Indeed, it wouldn't surprise me if, for that very reason, most of the consultants mentioned in this book don't even remember my name. I can only imagine how frustrating it must be for them to have to train up all the junior doctors, only to have to start from scratch just as their juniors have finally become halfway competent at performing their duties. I'd be lying if I said that this wasn't something that weighed on my mind as I walked onto the Cardiology ward on that first Monday in August.

Not long after I'd arrived, I was spotted by the aforementioned Dr Jackman. Enquiring as to who I was, I dutifully explained that I was one of the new juniors due to start on Wednesday, and wanted to come in and shadow the team for the day.

"And so you took it upon yourself to come in a day early? Hmm – we like that," he said, smiling wryly.

I couldn't help at that moment but feel ever-so-slightly smug. *I've impressed him*, I thought gleefully.

Unfortunately, it was possibly the last time I ever did.

Every consultant is different of course, but many of them do have one thing in common: they like to grill their juniors on clinical topics – ostensibly as a teaching tool, but also to help them gauge just how much their juniors know (or, indeed, don't). As ridiculous as it may sound, one of the greatest reliefs for me about no longer being a junior doctor is the knowledge that I will never again have to go through the painfully embarrassing process of being asked a difficult question by a senior – often in front of numerous colleagues – and then

14

wishing the world would swallow me whole as I'm forced to admit that I don't know the answer.

I understand why consultants do it. Rightly or wrongly, grilling the juniors has long been thought of as a way of motivating them to keep up to date with their knowledge, avoid becoming complacent and, ultimately, strive to be a better doctor. I have, however, always felt that certain consultants simply take this 'ritual' too far. Though it may work effectively as a motivator for some, I've personally felt strongly from day one (even going back to my days as a student) that being berated for a lack of knowledge only ever succeeds in making you feel humiliated, inadequate and disillusioned. Being made to feel like you're just not good enough is, to my mind, simply not a very good motivator.

To his credit, I don't ever recall Dr Jackman shouting at me (or, indeed, anyone else), and I never once considered him to be mean-spirited (unlike some of the consultants I later worked with – but more on them later). However, he did have a remarkable way of expressing his disappointment in you with just a furrow of his eyebrows and a wry smirk. He also had an inimitable way of letting you know that one of his clinical interrogations was coming.

Because the green team was aligned with Dr Jackman's yellow team, I was required to join Dr Jackman's Monday afternoon ward round each week – and there's no better opportunity for an educational cross-examination than on a ward round.

"So, Ahmed," Dr Jackman said enquiringly during our very first ward round together, "what are the defining characteristics of the fourth heart sound?" He then proceeded to adopt what I would later discover was his signature pose – moving his glasses down his nose, before folding his arms and fixing his piercing gaze upon me.

My heart sank (no pun intended). I hadn't the faintest idea what the answer was, and he knew it.

This was sadly a ritual that became all too common during my time in Cardiology – to the point that I rather began to loathe Monday afternoon ward rounds. Perhaps Dr Jackman's questions were excessively hard and probing, or perhaps my knowledge simply wasn't as good as it should have been. Either way, as much as I wanted to impress Dr Jackman, it wasn't something that I ever felt I succeeded in doing – barring perhaps that one fleeting moment on that very first Monday.

If there is an odd silver lining to my being grilled by Dr Jackman (always in his characteristic manner), it did lead to a rather amusing revelation. After one particularly gruelling ward round with him, one of the nurses came up to me, and I could instantly see that she had a look on her face akin to that of a love-struck schoolgirl.

"Erm, everything okay, Jo?" I asked bemusedly.

"Ooh, that Dr Jackman! I tell you, Ahmed – whenever he moves his glasses down his nose and folds those muscular arms of his… oof! I just go weak at the knees!"

It turned out that she wasn't alone. I subsequently discovered that pretty much each and every nurse on the ward was hopelessly and madly in love with this muscular, somewhat enigmatic, Kiwi inquisitor. Go figure.

CARRY ON CLERKING

No recollection of my time in Cardiology would be complete without mentioning Brenda, one of our ward clerks. A (shall we say) *rotund* woman in her fifties, Brenda is a character that I won't soon forget for two very good reasons: her blunt manner, and her *filthy* sense of humour.

Whatever else was going on in the department, Brenda could always be relied upon to tell it like it was – and, to be fair, she did it in such a way that made her very difficult to dislike. For the exact same reason, however, I was secretly relieved that her job didn't involve a great deal of patient contact. I shudder to think of the complaints her no-nonsense manner would doubtlessly invite.

Imagine my surprise then when I discovered about two months into the job that Brenda had, in fact, once been a nurse, before her growing realisation that she actually quite disliked patients made her decide to take up an administrative role instead. With this revelation predictably came some wonderful stories about Brenda's nursing heyday.

"Brenda," one of her nursing colleagues had enquired one day, "please could you help take Mrs Brookes to the toilet?" Mrs Brookes, I was told, was a woman with poorly controlled diabetes, who had recently had one of her feet amputated.

"Why?!," Brenda had replied in a shrill voice. "There's

nothing wrong with her other leg, is there? She can hop to the loo!"

On another occasion, Brenda was asked to give a sponge bath to a gentleman called Mr Salter, who had lost both of his legs during the Falklands War.

"Why?!," Brenda asked defiantly. "There's nothing wrong with his arms, is there? He can wash himself!"

So yes, tact, I quickly learned, was most definitely not Brenda's strong suit.

As part of her administrative role as a ward clerk, Brenda was responsible for ensuring that all patients went home with a discharge letter summarising their in-patient stay. These letters were all automatically saved to the patient's records, and were an invaluable resource for the GP, as well as if, for example, said patient ever ended up back in hospital.

One day, a patient (Mr Bools) was admitted onto the Cardiology ward who had previously been a 'guest' of ours around six months earlier. Will (the junior doctor for the blue team, whom I mentioned earlier) was trying to pull up the patient's previous discharge summary on the computer, but for some reason was struggling to do so.

A quick side note to this story: Will, I should mention, was a thoroughly lovely guy (who was very supportive of me throughout my Cardiology job), and – like Brenda – he had an irrepressible sense of humour. I remember once when Cameron (a mutual junior doctor colleague of ours) was locked out of the computer, and so asked Will if he could use his login ID until the issue was resolved.

"Sure thing – it's *will1982*," he replied.

"Thanks, mate. Sorry, and what's your password?"

Cameron asked.

Will lowered his head, smirked, and sheepishly replied, "It's *bollocks*. All lowercase."

But I digress...

When Will had finally given up on attempting to retrieve Mr Bools's old discharge letter, he asked Brenda to come over to the doctors' desk (which was in the middle of the ward) and give him a hand. Brenda then began suggesting possible solutions to Will as she stood over his shoulder and monitored the results. However, everything he tried failed to achieve the desired outcome.

After a solid five minutes of Will trying, and failing, to pull up the patient's letter, Brenda had clearly had enough. Frustrated, she suddenly cried out – in the middle of the ward, surrounded by a veritable swarm of doctors, nurses and patients: "What's wrong with you, Will?! You just can't get it up!"

As everyone within earshot began to burst out laughing, I was relieved to see that Will, now flashing his trademark cheeky smirk, saw the funny side.

"Brenda!", he exclaimed. "You can't say that! That's precisely the kind of statement that can wreck a man's confidence for ever, you know!"

My most abiding memory of Brenda, however, has got to be the time when we had a prison transfer patient on the ward. As the local prison was just a few miles down the road from the hospital, and given that we were the only specialist Cardiology unit in the region, such admissions were not uncommon.

When it came time for his discharge from hospital and back to prison, the patient, clad in distinctive orange overalls, was restrained in handcuffs and led away from his side room flanked by two male police officers. As he was escorted across the ward and towards the exit, the three men happened to pass by Brenda's office. Brenda had, in fact, been watching all this take place, an unmistakeable lust-filled look etched on her face as she practically drooled at the sight of this rather well-built felon.

Unable to resist, Brenda suddenly exclaimed, "Ooh, darling – be sure to save those handcuffs for me!"

Now, I don't know why this man was in prison (curious though I might've been, it was considered bad practice to ask – spoil sports). However, as a look of pure horror fell across the convict's face, I imagined that the prospect of once again being incarcerated safely behind bars – and away from the undressing eyes of this slightly mad, menopausal, middle-aged woman – had suddenly become hugely comforting to him.

COLOUR BLIND

Question: when you think of England, where does 'the North' end and 'the South' begin?

This is a question I have asked myself many times since I moved to the Midlands (what now feels like a lifetime ago). And I'm realising more and more that the answer simply depends on who you ask.

An extremely brief biography: I was born and brought up in East Anglia, the son of two Arabic doctors. When I was eighteen, I moved down to London to study medicine, and it was my intention to remain there when I started my foundation training (the term referring to a doctor's first two working years post-graduation). Life, however, had other plans.

The region (also known as a deanery) in London to which I applied during my final year of medical school was, it turned out, the most popular – and hence over-subscribed – deanery in the entire UK that year. And so it was that – just like those artillery models you see Generals indifferently pushing across a map during war room scenes in old black and white movies – I ended up unexpectedly being moved to the Midlands, some one hundred and fifty miles away from everyone and everything I knew. In the way that life is, however, being forced to move there turned out to be one of the best things that could've ever happened to me; not least of which because I ended up getting to know some incredible people, forming friendships that have lasted to this day, and meeting the woman who just over two years later became my wife.

That's not to say, however, that moving to the Midlands wasn't one hell of a culture shock (and if I'm honest, it still sometimes is). More than that, I suddenly felt when I moved there like I didn't really belong anywhere anymore. My London friends all started saying that I was now 'living up north', and to the people I encountered there I was most definitely (and still remain) a 'southerner'.

As I alluded to in the preface to this book, when you live in the Midlands you very quickly become accustomed to the lingo. 'Duck', 'shug', 'chick' – these, and many more, are all terms I suddenly started hearing on a daily basis. Somewhat embarrassingly, during my first few weeks as a doctor I was convinced that when people in hospital would (in their distinctive accent) call me 'duck', they were actually saying 'doc', as befitting what I now did for a living. It was only when I was referred to as 'duck' whilst out shopping in town that the penny finally dropped.

"How on earth could that shopkeeper possibly know I'm a doctor?" I mused. "*Ahh*, hang on..."

Worse still was a (much) later incident when the secretary for the Psychiatry consultant I worked for offered the following comment when she saw me removing a slightly worse-for-wear banana from my rucksack: "Ooh, I don't like the look of that narna!"

"I'm sorry, I don't quite follow," I replied, quite possibly sounding for all the world like the most ignorant southerner known to man.

"Your narna! I'm talking about your *narna*!" she replied exasperatedly.

It must've taken me a good ten seconds (not to mention the visual aid of her pointed finger) before I finally realised that she was talking about the slightly battered piece of fruit in my hands.

In time, the Midlands' slang actually became quite endearing, even if I did sometimes feel like I was living in a version of *Old MacDonald Had a Farm* ('with a *chick chick* here, and a *duck duck* there...'). Not all my colleagues appreciated this inimitable vernacular though, especially those who, like me, had been 'forcibly' relocated to this Brave New World, many miles from home. I remember one friend of mine (who, like me, was originally from East Anglia) reacting almost with abject horror when he was one day referred to as 'duck egg'.

"Duck egg? *Duck egg*?! What the hell does that even mean, Ahmed?? It's bollocks!"

As undoubtedly friendly as its people were, the city in which I now worked was admittedly not the most ethnically diverse of places, and as a person of Arabic descent this certainly led to some, shall we say, *interesting* conversations. The most memorable of these took place on none other than the Cardiology ward, about two months into my rotation.

I was writing in some patient notes when one of the nurses, Erica, suddenly appeared to notice me from the other end of the doctors' desk. Erica was, I should add, a woman who'd been born and raised in the city that I now called home. However, even knowing that, nothing could have possibly prepared me for the frankly bizarre line of questioning that was about to follow...

"Ahmed, I was just wondering. You're, erm, you're not from around here, are you?"

Wondering where on earth this was leading, I hesitantly replied, "Erm, no, no, I'm not."

Smacking her lips and pausing for a moment as she seemingly worked up the courage to ask the question which appeared to be burning on her mind, Erica tentatively continued, "Are you, erm... I mean, you're not *black*... are you?"

In an instant, I was suddenly overcome by two distinct emotions: incredulity (at the staggering ignorance behind the question), and amusement (at the sheer ridiculousness of the entire conversation). I also quickly realised that I had to be very diplomatic in my response. I was keen to ensure that it didn't come across as insulting to Erica (in spite of the stupidity of what she had just said), nor did I want my dismissal to sound so emphatic as to potentially come across as racist. Well, it was either that or just burst out laughing (and believe me, it took all my resolve not to). In the end, I replied with what I feel was a very measured response:

"Erm, no Erica – I'm Arabic."

Adding to the utter incomprehension of Erica's question was that one of the other junior doctors on the ward, a man named Daikun, was of Nigerian descent. So how exactly could Daikun and I *both* be black in Erica's eyes? This was something I never quite figured out. Maybe Erica just had really poor eyesight?

Having just name-dropped him, I couldn't possibly close out

this chapter without talking about the truly fascinating man that was Daikun: the great enigma.

Over the course of our four months together in Cardiology, Daikun would periodically reveal a previously unknown nugget of information about himself, and his unique backstory. It transpired that Daikun was once a consultant Cardiologist in his native Nigeria, and had even been part of the private medical team that served one of that nation's monarchs. Ultimately though, for reasons unknown, Daikun had been forced from his homeland as a political refugee, under threat of violent (perhaps even lethal) retribution from the regime that he had once so loyally served. And so it was that he ended up in the Midlands, forced to slum it once again as a junior doctor, and work his way back up the proverbial food chain to regain the senior position he had once held. But did any of that hardship dent his confidence, or subdue his outgoing personality? Not at all. Indeed, in the relatively short amount of time he had been in the UK, Daikun had established an impressive social life that would undoubtedly be the envy of many. He drove around everywhere in a top-of-the-line sports car. He spent his weekends down in London, hitting the clubs and picking up attractive women. He was even close personal friends with a then top name premiere league footballer.

Before long though, my colleagues and I were astounded by an even more incredible fact: almost the entirety of Daikun's story was, in short, a load of bollocks.

Ultimately, Daikun's flare for exaggeration became his undoing. As the improbabilities in his stories continued to mount, huge and glaring inconsistencies began appearing. It doubtless didn't help that Daikun also had the unfortunate habit of often contradicting himself when recounting his extravagant tales. It wasn't long, therefore, before we were all forced to conclude that the majority, if not the entirety, of Daikun's remarkable backstory was simply a massive lie (though I think it's safe to assume that he was indeed from Nigeria). The whole situation couldn't help but remind me of a classic line from the first *Austin Powers* film, spoken by Dr Evil: 'My father would womanise, he would drink... he would make outrageous claims, like he invented the question mark'.

The subject of classic comedy films also brings to mind another curious fact about Daikun. Whenever I would go to the doctors' mess – our designated rest area, of sorts – I would invariably see Daikun there as well. Typically, he could be seen lounging on one of the sofas, chatting to one of the other doctors, an unfamiliar gentleman who was also of African descent. One day, I asked my Cardiology colleague, Sarah, who Daikun's companion was.

"I'm not a hundred percent sure, actually," Sarah replied. "I always hear Daikun refer to him as his 'brother', but I don't know whether he means an actual brother, or if he just says that because they're both black." As I heard these words, I couldn't help but hear echoes of the eponymous (and loveably empty-headed) hero from the film *Zoolander*, who spoke the following words at the joint funeral for three of his friends: 'Rufus, Brint and Meekus were like brothers to me. And when I say brother, I don't mean, like, an actual brother – but I mean it like the way black people use it. Which is more meaningful, I think'.

As if his talent for exaggeration/blatant lying wasn't enough, Daikun also holds another distinction for me: he is, without a doubt, the single laziest doctor I've ever met (which explains why he spent the majority of his time in the doctors' mess). By the end of our time in Cardiology, Daikun's ability to shirk work and somehow get away with just doing the bare minimum had become nothing short of legendary.

One of the junior doctors' on call responsibilities in Cardiology was to 'clerk in' patients who were admitted onto the ward the evening before they were due to have an elective (i.e. planned) procedure. This would involve, as a minimum, taking a history from the patient (detailing key facts such as their symptoms, medical history, current medications, etc.), examining them, and then formulating a management plan that adequately incorporated any essential pre-procedure requirements.

Whenever Daikun was on call overnight, he would always wait until late in the evening before clerking in these elective patients – and it quickly became apparent to all of us why. Essentially, Daikun waited until the patient fell asleep in order to be able to carry out one of the quickest, most slap dash clerkings known to man. A 'Daikun special' was, for all the wrong reasons, truly a marvel to behold. The history section would be copied entirely from the patient's last outpatient clinic letter, the examination section would often simply state, 'patient not examined as sleeping', and the management plan section would typically read, 'plan as per last clinic letter'.

Unsurprisingly, Daikun's laissez faire attitude very quickly began to rub people up the wrong way; after all, if he wasn't doing the work, then that meant someone else had to pick up the slack, regardless of how much work they had on themselves. But karma always catches up with you in the end.

At the end of each hospital rotation, junior doctors have to ask their colleagues to complete something called a 360 degree assessment for them, an online form that allows said colleague to give anonymised feedback on that doctor's performance. These forms are then collated to form part of the doctor's next educational supervisor review. In hospitals, you would need a minimum of ten responses before the mandatory assessment is considered complete. Recipients of the 360 degree forms, however, are under no formal obligation to complete them.

Again, not surprisingly given his workshy attitude, the other junior doctors on the ward weren't exactly lining up to fill in 360 degree assessments for Daikun – and, as the end of our four-month attachment neared, his failure to secure the ten completed feedback forms he needed caused Daikun to panic. Fortunately, he had a plan to deal with this. Unfortunately, that plan involved me.

"Ahmed," Daikun piped up cheerily one Friday afternoon, as I gathered my belongings from the staffroom and prepared to head home for the day. "Would you please kindly complete a 360 degree assessment for me? I need it doing before we change over next Wednesday."

"Sure, Daikun," I replied, "no problem." I had the distinct feeling in that moment that Daikun had only asked me to do this simply because he had no one else left to ask. He and I hadn't really worked together much over the preceding four months and, to be frank, I didn't really have many positive things to say about the guy. However, I was young, and eager to please, and knew deep down that I wouldn't have the heart to write anything negative about this man, which could end up being damaging for his next appraisal. And I think Daikun knew that.

That weekend, I was so busy I completely forgot to complete Daikun's 360 degree assessment. Fortunately though, he was more than happy to give me a reminder or three once Monday arrived.

No sooner had I hung up my jacket in the staffroom on Monday morning when I heard the door open behind me and a somewhat disapproving voice call out, "Ahmed – you have not completed my 360 degree assessment. Please can you do it as soon as possible? It's very important."

"Yes, of course Daikun. I'm so sorry; it just completely slipped my mind at the weekend, but I promise I'll fill it in today."

Unmoved, Daikun replied, "Okay, but please make sure you do it."

Several busy hours later, I was back in the staffroom at lunchtime in order to pick up my jacket so I could grab a quick sandwich from the canteen. It wasn't long before I heard the familiar, and now rather stern, voice emanating from behind me.

"Ahmed – I've just checked, and you have still not completed my 360 degree assessment. Please can you do it as soon as possible?"

Was he serious? Didn't he realise I was doing him a pretty big favour (and somewhat against my better judgement)? Also, when exactly was I supposed to have found the time to do his form during what had been a particularly hectic morning? It wasn't, however, much of a stretch to imagine that Daikun had probably spent the vast majority of *his* morning sat at a computer screen, periodically clicking refresh on his online appraisal portfolio, eagerly hoping to see the number of completed 360 degree forms increase by one.

When replying, my tone of voice failed to mask some of my underlying frustration and bewilderment. "Yes, Daikun. I promised I'd complete your form, and I will. But it isn't really feasible for me to do it while we're at work – I'll do it as soon as I get home tonight."

"Okay, but please make sure you do. It's very important."

When I did finally get home that evening, my first order of business was simple: log into my e-mails and fill in Daikun's stupid form – if nothing else, for the sake of an easy life. Waiting for me in my inbox was an e-mail from none other than Daikun, sent just an hour earlier.

'Ahmed', it read, 'I've just checked, and you have still not completed my 360 degree assessment. You need to do this as soon as possible. It's very important'.

Believe me when I say that I have never, before or since, done such a thoroughly half-arsed job of completing a feedback form as I did when filling in Daikun's assessment. Though given the person to whom it related, I suppose that's oddly fitting.

PART II

VASCULAR SURGERY

TAKING THE "FUN" OUT OF DYSFUNCTIONAL

For most junior doctors, FY1 is divided up into three, four-month rotations: one medical, one surgical, and one 'other'. And so it was that, after my four months in Cardiology were up, I moved onto vascular surgery – a strong contender for the worst of the nine hospital-based jobs I completed during my time as a junior doctor.

What was it that made that surgical attachment such a negative experience? Was it the hours (which were long and punishing)? Was it the gruelling on call schedule? Was it the pervading sense of inefficiency and disorganisation in the way that things were run on the wards? It was, in fact, none of these things (though they certainly didn't help). I'm even prepared to overlook the fact that, on one frustrating occasion, I had £40 in cash stolen from my wallet whilst it sat 'safely' inside my jacket, which was hung up behind the locked staffroom door – thus making the prospect of the money having been stolen by one of the other doctors or nurses a highly likely and unsettling possibility. No, what made my time in surgery such a misery was, quite simply, the surgeons.

Around the time I started the rotation, a rumour began spreading amongst the junior doctors that the six consultants who made up the upper tier of our vascular surgery department were so reviled by their surgical peers working at nearby hospitals that they had been dubbed 'psychotic'. Though none of the consultants thankfully turned out to be axe murderers (at least not as far as I know), it was a label I soon discovered wasn't far off the mark.

There is a well-worn cliché concerning surgeons, which is that they're brash, arrogant and rude individuals, with a massive God complex, appalling people skills and even worse tempers. Whilst I can't speak for surgeons everywhere, of course, these ones most certainly fitted the surgical cliché to a tee. And sadly, this wasn't just true of the consultants, but most of their registrars as well.

In order for me to give this part of the story proper context, it's important that I mention that my time in vascular surgery was also coloured by a major event in my personal life. About a month into the attachment, my mother died. She had been ill for some time, though I had chosen (for a variety of reasons) not to tell anyone at work that she was unwell. In the days immediately before and after she passed away though, I had no choice but to tell the department what was happening, so that I could be excused from work on compassionate grounds to be at home with my mum and my family.

When I returned to work (after a total of seven days' absence), I was truly touched by the outpouring of kindness, sympathy and support from my fellow FY1 doctors. However, out of all the Vascular consultants and registrars, only one of them (Mr Deepak) actually took the time to approach me to say he was sorry to hear about my mother, and check if I was holding up okay. The rest of them never even said a word –

and, I'll admit, that stung.

What hurt even worse was when my new nominated clinical supervisor, an Irish woman called Ms Hartigan (and the only female Vascular consultant on the team), marked my progress as 'unsatisfactory' in my mandatory mid-rotation report, which was completed approximately four weeks after my return from compassionate leave. Her report read:

'Ahmed is clinically competent, but does not work to the standards of efficiency that I would expect of an FY1 doctor. However, I note that he has recently suffered a personal bereavement, and imagine that this may have been playing on his mind in recent weeks'.

Yeah? Well no shit, Sherlock. Clearly, Ms Hartigan was wasted as a surgeon, when she so obviously should have been a Psychiatrist instead.

Reading that report cut deep. Not helping matters was the fact that Ms Hartigan didn't even grant me the courtesy of telling me in advance (as is customary practice) that she was going to mark my progress as unsatisfactory. My boss not expressing any kind of condolences for my mum's passing was one thing, but the somewhat underhand way she went about this 'surprise' negative evaluation just seemed cruel. I'd be lying if I said my pride wasn't dented by reading that report; like most of my FY1 colleagues, I had always been a bit of a 'swot' at school, a straight A student who had never once received a grade of 'unsatisfactory progress' in all my life.

Thankfully – spoiler alert – I did manage to turn things around before the end of my time in vascular surgery (at least in Ms Hartigan's eyes), and was given that all-important grade of 'satisfactory progress' in my end-of-rotation report.

And though I wasn't ever her biggest fan, I never really had a major problem with Ms Hartigan (her mid-rotation report aside). As Vascular surgeons go, she was still very much on the tamer end of the scale. I even found amusement in some of her mannerisms. Ms Hartigan was someone who often became surprisingly expressive when describing patients she had seen, or recounting a surgical procedure she had just performed. On one occasion, I recall her saying (in her distinctive Irish brogue), "So then I pulled back the sheet, took one look at the patient's foot, and said to myself – *yeeesh*! I don't like the look of that foot!"

However, whilst Ms Hartigan could perhaps be classed as mostly harmless (even if she's never going to win any awards for empathy), the same most definitely cannot be said about the majority of her colleagues – a veritable rogues' gallery of individuals, whose personalities and interpersonal skills left an awful lot to be desired.

HOW BLACK WAS MY JACKET

Before I get on to the rest of the consultants, I must first give an 'honourable' mention to two of their registrars: Mr Wilkerson and Mr Prabath. Incidentally, if you've ever been curious as to why surgeons are referred to as Mr/Mrs rather than Dr (and I have discovered over the years – sometimes to my peril – that some surgeons are *very* particular about this; they *earned* that Mr/Mrs, thank you very much), it's an homage to the fact that the very first surgeons were actually barbers and butchers. This is (you perhaps won't be surprised to hear) a fact that crossed my mind many times during my stint in vascular surgery (and later in Orthopaedics).

Mr Steven Wilkerson was a man who strode onto the ward every morning wearing the same black jacket and the same slightly pained look on his face that practically screamed he'd much rather be somewhere – *anywhere* – else. And before long, I discovered why (though the jacket I'll just have to chalk up to a somewhat questionable fashion choice).

I think it's fair to say that most career surgeons don't really feel invigorated at work unless they're in the operating theatre, actually doing what it is they got into surgery to do – i.e. cutting people open and fixing things (a gross oversimplification, of course, but one that's still apt). As a result, dealing with talking, *conscious* patients in outpatient clinics or on ward rounds isn't really most surgeons' forte, with many viewing such commitments as simply barriers (albeit necessary ones) to actually getting to theatre and doing what it is they love. Additionally, for more junior surgeons in particular, getting as much time in theatre as possible is not only desirable, but essential if you want to gain more experience, hone your skills and, ultimately, advance up the highly competitive surgical career ladder.

Mr Wilkerson was certainly one such hungry young career surgeon, who preferred to spend as much time in theatre as possible. However, in vascular surgery, every morning would begin the same way (come rain or shine): the ward round. Twice a week, this would be led by one of the consultants, which meant that on the other days that responsibility would instead fall to one of the registrars. However, every minute spent on the wards meant a minute less operating, and so the registrars therefore did their utmost to ensure that the ward round was completed as quickly as humanly possible. Mr Wilkerson was undoubtedly the worst offender when it came to this, and I soon came to understand that the dejected look on his face when he and his black jacket walked onto the ward just before 8:00 was unsubtle code for 'Come on, let's get this over with'.

On any given day, our team would be responsible for around thirty–forty surgical patients, often spread out over at least four or five different wards. The patients consisted of a mixture of pre and post-op patients (plus those being managed non-surgically), and turnaround was *fast*. But still, every one of them had to be seen on the daily ward round. Frankly, trying to keep up with who all the patients were, where they each were, what they had come into hospital with, what operation(s) they had had (if any), what their latest test results were, etc. was an almost Herculean task, made all the more difficult by the fact that – though there were nominally four FY1 doctors working in vascular surgery – one or two of us would invariably be away on a given day (on call or on leave). If one of the patients became seriously unwell, looking after them would inevitably take up a large chunk of your day. And on top of everything else, the ward nurses – who, to be fair, were often just as stretched and overwhelmed as the junior doctors – were never shy about reminding us if a drug chart needed rewriting or a patient's discharge paperwork had yet to be completed. Though such responsibilities are hardly confined to vascular surgery (or indeed surgery in general), I must confess that my abiding memory of those four months remains running from ward to ward like a headless chicken, and persistently fighting against the nagging fear that I was way out of my depth, and slowly drowning.

Ostensibly, there were two other doctors in vascular surgery (both of whom were second year so-called core surgical trainees) who were supposed to help out the FY1 doctors on the wards: Farah and Mustafa. However, they were almost always to be found in theatre as well, and – to make matters worse – just three weeks into the rotation, Mustafa was forced to abruptly leave his post when it was discovered his UK work visa was invalid. When Cindy, his replacement, finally started work a mere two months later, she made it clear from day one that she was *not* prepared to help out with any of the 'menial' ward jobs; as she so eloquently put it, "I've been the ward bitch already – that's your job now." As you can tell, Cindy was a real charmer.

Ironically, one of the main ideas behind doing the daily surgical ward round is to try to bring a sense of order to all this chaos, by working as a team to review each patient, and ensure that a (senior-led) plan has been put in place for that person's ongoing treatment and/or discharge. I quickly understood, however, that for practical reasons (given the sheer number of patients under your team's care, not to mention the full patient list waiting to be operated on in theatre that day), surgical ward rounds had to be quick. That being said, I don't think anything could have prepared me for the sheer breakneck speed of Mr Wilkerson's rounds, not one of which ever lasted much beyond forty-five minutes. To put that into perspective, I've done some medical jobs where the ward round (often seeing significantly fewer patients than on surgical rounds) lasted up to *seven hours*, essentially leaving little time for anything else that day! In short, a Mr Wilkerson ward round was an exercise in chaos.

With any surgical rounds, you learn very quickly that you have to be on the ball. If you don't come prepared, and don't keep up, you'll soon be hopelessly lost. Mr Wilkerson's ward rounds, however, were a step beyond. No sooner would you arrive at the patient's bedside, find the right page in the notes, and get hold of the observation chart (having scarcely more than a few moments to actually look at it), before Mr Wilkerson curtly barked his plan at you – often just the word 'home' – and moved onto the next patient. Frankly, as awful and unprofessional as it sounds, there were some days I didn't even bother closing the curtains around a patient's bed when Mr Wilkerson came to review them. After all, there seemed barely any point, since you'd just have to open them again mere moments later (sometimes literally as soon as you'd finished closing them). There were even days when Mr Wilkerson would declare just prior to starting the round, "Don't bother bringing the notes this morning – that'll just take up time. Write in them later." All in all, under Mr Wilkerson's stewardship the average amount of time spent with each patient on a ward round was typically less than sixty seconds.

Think about that for a moment: if your relative had just had major surgery and was being reviewed the following morning, how reassured would you feel knowing that the surgeon in charge had spent under a minute assessing their fitness to go home? As I have sadly learned from personal experience in the years since, once you know what goes on behind the scenes, it can be an especially disconcerting experience when a loved one falls ill and you find yourself back on the other, non-medical side of the fence.

This haphazard, rushed style of reviewing surgical patients must have inevitably left many of them feeling unimportant, or even uncared for. I remember all too well the looks of frustration or puzzlement on many patients' faces as Hurricane Ward Round swept through the patient bays, leaving a trail of sheer bewilderment in its wake. This approach was bad enough when the patients were stable, and being earmarked for discharge home; however, when things were more complicated (and especially if the surgeon had to impart some bad news) it could be an unmitigated disaster.

I wrote earlier that surgeons are not typically well-known for their expert communication skills, and there was no clearer example of this than Mr Wilkerson. I vividly remember a surgical patient called Barbara, a lady in her sixties, who had been admitted with a rare but serious condition called necrotizing fasciitis (also known, grimly, as flesh-eating disease), in which a bacterial infection results in the destruction of the body's soft tissues. In Barbara's case, the infection had – over the course of several weeks – slowly yet progressively caused the soft tissues of her left arm to waste away. Sadly, multiple courses of potent antibiotics, as well as maggot therapy (yes, really; this is, nauseatingly, exactly what it sounds like – and no, I couldn't believe this was actually still practised in western medicine in the twenty-first century either), had failed to halt the advance of Barbara's necrotizing fasciitis, and this had unhappily left the surgical team with just one treatment option: a below-shoulder amputation.

To Barbara's great misfortune, it was Mr Wilkerson whose job it was to break the devastating news to her on the ward round. And he did about as bad a job of it as you could possibly imagine.

"Look, Barbara", he began matter-of-factly, "I don't think it'll come as any surprise to you that we're just not winning the battle against your infection here. And so I'm afraid that arm's gonna have to come off."

A stunned silence filled the room.

Barbara, obviously, was devastated – who wouldn't be? What I'll never forget though, was the look of shock still visibly etched on her face through the tears that followed Mr Wilkerson's appallingly delivered bombshell, and the moment she then looked up at him, her lip aquiver, and softly uttered the words, "I can't believe you just said it like that."

Mr Wilkerson, looking to all the world at that moment

like he was simply incapable of empathy or basic human decency, offered a pathetically weak, "Sorry", before leaving the patient's room (I thank God that Barbara was at least in a side room when this fumbled bombshell was delivered, and not one of the patient bays), going up to one of the nurses, and indifferently asking, "Can someone get Barbara a cup of tea, please? She's a little upset."

I'd like to be able to tell you that, despite Mr Wilkerson not having the best rapport with his patients (Barbara, quite rightly, gave him the evil eye for months after their life-altering conversation), he was at least very supportive of his juniors. This, sadly, wasn't the case either.

On one occasion, I was clerking in a patient who had just been admitted to the surgical ward. When I felt the gentleman's abdomen (as part of my routine examination) it had a very odd consistency to it that I had not previously ever come across when feeling someone's tummy. In short, though I realise it's hardly the most scientific word, his tummy felt lumpy. Unsure as to the significance of this (if any), I decided to ask one of my seniors for advice. Unluckily for me, the senior who happened to be on the ward was Mr Wilkerson.

When I, somewhat hesitantly, relayed the story to him, he gave me possibly the biggest smirk I'd ever seen break out across someone's face, before eventually, if highly reluctantly, agreeing to quickly review the patient. Thankfully, the 'lumpy' feel of the patient's abdomen was ultimately nothing to be concerned about (he had previously been a recreational drug user, and the lumps were areas of scar tissue from where he had injected himself). However, Mr Wilkerson spent the rest of the day bemoaning the all-of-three minutes I had taken up of his time to review the patient. Indeed, when the two of us re-emerged from the patient's side room, and a fellow registrar asked Mr Wilkerson where he had just been, he replied derisively, "I've just been in to examine a man who Ahmed reckoned had a *funny tummy*."

A few weeks later, another of the patients on our ward developed a haematoma (a collection of blood) over his right arm. Complicating matters was the fact that the gentleman in question was a kidney dialysis patient, and his haematoma had come up right next to his arteriovenous fistula (a connection between an artery and a vein that is sometimes – as in that patient's case – created surgically for the purposes of dialysis).

Mr Wilkerson breezed onto the ward one afternoon (black jacket present and correct), having been bleeped (i.e. paged) by one of the nurses about the haematoma. Spotting me, he promptly asked me to fetch him the necessary surgical drainage kit (including a large syringe and needle), and then bring it to the patient's bedside.

"Do you need any help with the haematoma drainage, Mr Wilkerson?", I asked.

After a brief contemplative pause, he replied, "You know what? Why don't you do it, Ahmed? I'll come and assist you."

What followed was, quite possibly, one of the most nerve-wracking ten minutes of my entire life.

After we had set up all the equipment, ready to go, Mr Wilkerson turned to me and said, "Now remember, Ahmed, the haematoma is really near this gentleman's fistula. If you push the needle in too far, you'll hit it – and that wouldn't be good."

Why Mr Wilkerson chose to remind me of this fact (of

which I was already well aware) now, moments before I was about to insert the needle, and in front of the patient to boot (who was now clued into the fact that I had obviously never done this procedure before) I will never know.

In those excruciatingly tense next few moments, as I prepared to insert the needle (with Mr Wilkerson unhelpfully breathing down my neck, and the patient gazing up at me with silent panic), I honestly couldn't hear a pin drop. It later dawned on me that this was essentially a real-life game of Operation, only in this case my patient was an actual human being, and the stakes if I messed up were so much higher than a simple irritating *bzzzt*.

Thankfully, the procedure appeared to go well, and I watched with relief as the haematoma slowly began to shrink. Less confidence-inspiring was Mr Wilkerson feeling the need to lean in every few minutes and whisper, "Remember, you're really near the fistula."

When I arrived on the ward the next day, Mr Wilkerson was, unusually, already there. As soon as he saw me, a grim look crossed his face, and he said exasperatedly, "Ahmed, that patient whose haematoma you drained yesterday has just been rushed into theatre. His haemoglobin dropped massively overnight!"

As I looked at Mr Wilkerson, racked with guilt and lost for words, he suddenly broke out in a huge grin and said, "Ha! No, not really! Only joking – the man's fine."

Sadly, this wasn't the only time Mr Wilkerson played this 'hilarious' game with me. Some weeks after haematoma-gate, I was assisting Mr Wilkerson in theatre, and was given the opportunity to 'close up' at the end of surgery. The following day, Mr Wilkerson approached me on the ward, that familiar grimace on his face.

"Ahmed, you know Mrs Henry, the lady we operated on yesterday? Those stitches you put in came apart when she was in recovery, and I had to re-suture her wound from scratch; it was a *mess*." And then, somewhat predictably, came the 'reveal' moments later. "Ha! No, not really! Only joking – the lady's fine."

Probity was, it must be said, not always Mr Wilkerson's strong suit. I remember on one occasion sheepishly having to explain to him that the chest x-ray request I had put through for one of the pre-op inpatients (simply because, per local departmental protocol, almost all Vascular patients had a routine chest x-ray prior to their operation) had been rejected by Radiology because I'd made the mistake of being honest and writing "Pre-op chest x-ray" on the request form. Radiology had not considered that a good enough reason to expose the patient in question to x-ray radiation, especially if she had absolutely no chest symptoms – and I can't say I blamed them. With a scowl on his face, and without missing a beat, Mr Wilkerson picked up the ward phone, rang Radiology, and proceeded to spin an outrageously tall tale about how this patient was complaining of fevers, shortness of breath and a cough. An hour later, she got her chest x-ray.

Is that kind of lie justifiable? I suppose that's debatable, depending on the circumstances. Even the more junior core surgical trainees were not immune from being creative with the truth. I remember one of them once impersonating a consultant and ringing up the hospital catering department to put in a complaint, after one of the patients grumbled during the ward round that he was missing his favourite dish: sausage and mash. Unbelievably, it was then brought down to the patient within fifteen minutes! In Mr Wilkerson's case, however, he lied with the kind of smug arrogance that made you question just how altruistic his motives really were.

Whilst it's perhaps not the most noble thing for me to admit, I must confess to an immense sense of personal satisfaction when I witnessed Mr Wilkerson make a bit of a fool of himself not long before the end of my four-month rotation.

Often, consultants are happy leaving the more minor or routine surgical procedures in the hands of their registrars. To be honest, I have always suspected that most registrars much prefer to be left to their own devices in theatre, partly because it gives them more hands-on experience, but mainly because it means that they don't then have to indulge in that other great surgical cliché: sucking up to the boss. Whilst many surgeons may consider themselves to be alpha males, even they can become surprisingly demure when the leader of the pack turns up.

One morning, Mr Wilkerson was given his own surgical list, consisting of three or four fairly routine operations. One of these procedures was a cholecystectomy (the surgical removal of the gallbladder). As Mr Wilkerson was short-staffed in theatre that day, I was drafted in to assist him.

Everything was going well, and we had just reached the point in the operation where the cystic duct (the tube that drains the gallbladder) needed to be cut. A cholecystectomy is typically done via so-called keyhole surgery, and involves the use of video to help guide your actions. In short, it's delicate work.

Literally just as Mr Wilkerson was preparing to cut the cystic duct, Ms Hartigan suddenly walked into theatre, and loudly enquired (in that unmistakeable Irish twang), "How's it going, Steve?"

Momentarily distracted, Mr Wilkerson's hand suddenly slipped, and he accidentally cut open a large hole in the gallbladder itself, bile oozing voluminously from within (all captured on the surgical equivalent of CCTV).

Ms Hartigan was visibly unimpressed.

Did this slip-up in any way put the patient at harm? No. After all, the gallbladder was just about to be taken out anyway, so poking a hole in it at this stage would not have been in any way dangerous. It is, however, pretty embarrassing, especially for a career surgeon who's eager to look good in front of the boss. Without a doubt, I had never before seen Mr Wilkerson so flustered and red-faced.

Saying this may be neither big nor clever, but my God, the smug prat deserved it. In that moment, Barbara (the lady who'd had the necrotizing fasciitis) crossed my mind, and I really felt like calling out to one of the theatre staff and saying, "Can someone get Steve a cup of tea, please? He's a little upset."

BETWEEN THE EYES

The other Vascular registrar I have to mention, Mr Kapil Prabath, is someone whom I never quite got a handle on. On the one hand, he was a generally upbeat individual, with a quick wit and an unmistakeable twinkle in his eye. Personality-wise, he couldn't have been more different to the perennially dour Mr Wilkerson, with said contrast even extending to his dress sense. A world away from that tired-looking black jacket, Mr Prabath was renowned for his bright (think frequently pink with stripes) shirts, which even led to his juniors coining the Lloyd Webber-inspired phrase, 'Kapil and his amazing technicolour work shirt'.

On the other hand, Mr Prabath was also not immune to some of the negative surgical stereotypes I referred to earlier, one of which being his (sometimes very dark) sense of humour.

A quick side note: I've touched on workplace-based humour already in this book, and for me its importance shouldn't be understated. Don't get me wrong, it's obviously a very serious job that doctors do – we literally deal with life and death on a daily basis, and I have always prided myself on never poking fun at a patient's expense; it's part of the reason why (as I stated in the preface) I consciously chose to make the focus of this book the (frequently oddball) colleagues I worked with during my time as a junior doctor, rather than the people who entrust their health – and very lives – into our hands. However, because of how serious this job can be, I've always felt that you sometimes need a bit of levity to prevent the work from totally draining you emotionally. In short, it helps keep you sane.

Medical humour is definitely an acquired taste; surgical humour even more so. As an example, I remember one occasion when I was sat on the ward with two of my other junior doctor colleagues. We were suddenly approached by a very morose-looking Mr Deepak (one of the Vascular consultants).

"Hi, guys. Have you seen Mr Prabath around?"

"No, Mr Deepak," my colleague Rebecca replied. "Not since the ward round this morning, I'm afraid."

"Yes," Mr Deepak sombrely replied, before adding with an almost macabre flourish, "that's because he's *dead*."

And with that, Mr Deepak promptly left the ward without another word, leaving three very confused-looking juniors in his wake. Mr Deepak had obviously been joking (his sense of humour was also known to be jet black at times), but honestly? I just didn't think that kind of thing was actually funny.

Coming back to Mr Prabath, if his loud technicolour work shirts weren't evidence enough, subtlety, it must be said, was not always his forte when it came to humour. A perfect example of this is an offhand comment he once made to me in theatre.

To give you some context, for many years now I have had a beard. I have learned the hard way not to grow it too long as it then begins to look less wannabe-hipster and more (as my family have often remarked) 'religious'. For a man of Arabic descent such as myself, having a so-called religious beard is not always an enviable proposition; indeed, my late mum, in an uncharacteristic display of blunt candour, once even said, "You can't go walking around on the London underground with your beard looking like that – you'll get shot." My brother took a slightly different (though no less subtle) tack when letting me know his opinion on my facial fuzz, one day affixing a photo of disgraced radical Islamic cleric (or mullah) Abu Hamza al-Masri to my bedroom door. Point taken.

One Tuesday afternoon, I was drafted in to assist both Mr Prabath and Mr Wilkerson in theatre. It just so happened that through laziness and lack of time I'd unintentionally let my beard grow out a bit. At one point during the operation, I was assisting the registrars by applying the local anaesthetic drug Lidocaine to a part of the surgical wound, using a syringe.

"Ahmed," Mr Wilkerson said, "there's no need to be so delicate. You have to be a bit more liberal with your use of the Lidocaine."

With a loud guffaw, Mr Prabath suddenly chimed in, "Liberal? *Ahmed*? Come on, Steve, just take a look at that beard – he's a mullah!"

I later relayed this particular story to my FY1 colleague, Marcus, opining that with my beard still not being overly long, I was surely, at best, only Mullah Light. With a retort that still baffles me to this day, he fired back:

"Well, Ahmed, I'd actually say you were more Mullah Fruit Corner."

Ultimately, I found Mr Prabath's mullah comment harmless and inoffensive. What is not defensible, however, was a later incident involving the registrar, which shocked me as few have done before or since. When I reflect now, some years later, on what transpired, I'm still not entirely certain how Mr Prabath got away with his actions without having to face some kind of disciplinary hearing.

The event in question centred on an elderly patient called Mrs Watson. She suffered from attacks of pseudoseizures (fits that, though often misdiagnosed as being due to epilepsy, are actually typically psychological in origin, usually due to emotional distress). Mrs Watson had a number of pseudoseizures during her time with us on the ward. Due to the characteristic way in which her hands would jerk from side to side during an attack, Mr Prabath decided to bestow upon the patient the rather cruel moniker 'Jazz Hands Watson'.

One morning, Mr Prabath and I happened to be on the ward when one of the nurses, Vanessa, approached and informed us that Mrs Watson was having another pseudoseizure. Mr Prabath then promptly walked over to the patient's bed (myself in tow) and drew back the curtains to the sight of Mrs Watson having a full-on fit. It was the first time Mr Prabath had actually witnessed one of the patient's non-epileptic attacks.

Unperturbed, Mr Prabath turned to Vanessa and calmly asked her for a ten millilitre syringe filled with water. Vanessa appeared visibly puzzled, but dutifully headed towards the ward's storeroom in order to oblige the registrar's odd request. In fairness, Vanessa was not the only one who was confused in that moment. There is no specific drug treatment for pseudoseizures (essentially you just need to wait for them to stop on their own), and so I genuinely had no idea what Mr Prabath had in mind. And even if he was planning to administer some kind of medication to try to arrest Mrs Watson's fit, then why ask for the syringe to be filled with just water?

I soon got my answer.

Vanessa swiftly returned, and gingerly handed the water-filled syringe to Mr Prabath. To the sound of stunned silence, Mr Prabath then suddenly pointed the syringe at Mrs Watson's face, before squirting her with its entire contents at point-blank range.

The patient stopped fitting in an instant, a visible look of shock on her face (which surely belied the thought, "*What did he just do*?!"), before her pseudoseizure resumed a few moments later.

"See?" Mr Prabath exclaimed, almost triumphantly. "I knew she wasn't having a proper seizure!"

Without another word (and with Vanessa and myself both unable to offer any of our own), Mr Prabath returned to the doctors' desk before proceeding to document in Mrs Watson's notes. Undeniably curious, I couldn't help but take a look at the poor lady's notes as soon as Mr Prabath had left the ward, wondering what on earth his written justification would be for essentially turning a syringe into a Super Soaker and using it on a patient:

Mr Prabath, surgical registrar

Asked to attend the patient's bedside by staff nurse Vanessa at 11:20 a.m. – pseudoseizure witnessed.

And that was it, the entirety of his written entry, with not a single mention of Mr Prabath's trigger-happy behaviour. I guess I shouldn't have been all that surprised.

Mr Prabath wasn't the only member of our team who clearly struggled with how best to document one of Mrs Watson's witnessed pseudoseizures. Another of my junior doctor colleagues, Marcus, was asked to see Mrs Watson just two days later during another of her pseudoseizures. His method of choice was to try to stop her fit by applying what's called a sternal rub, which involves rubbing a patient's breastbone with a closed fist in order to assess their responsiveness. His subsequent documentation, I'll admit, was somewhat unorthodox:

I observed the patient having a pseudoseizure at 2:45 p.m. I applied a gentle sternal rub, and Mrs Watson suddenly looked up at me and said, "What?!"

Dr Marcus Johansson, FY1

What really threw me, however, was a conversation I overheard between Mr Prabath and a fellow surgical registrar that occurred just a few short hours after the infamous 'squirt gate' incident.

"Ben, you'll never guess what. You know Jazz Hands Watson, the pseudoseizure lady on ward C3? This morning I squirted her in the face with some water to stop her from fitting," before adding proudly, "Got her right between the eyes!"

Mr Prabath and his colleague then both started laughing raucously. Any respect I'd had for the man vanished in an instant.

Losing respect for Mr Prabath genuinely saddened me, as (flashes of clichéd surgical machismo aside) he really had come across as a nice guy, and he was unquestionably supportive and approachable in a way that very few others within that particular team were. However, the incident with Mrs Watson couldn't help but make me look at him in a different light. Yet what truly solidified the change in how I viewed him was the way he treated my colleague, Farah.

Farah was, as I mentioned earlier, one of the core surgical trainees with us in vascular surgery. This meant she was part of the specialty surgical training scheme, and thus on the training ladder towards becoming a fully-fledged surgeon. However, whilst she was more senior than myself and the other FY1s (you can only actually be accepted onto a specialty training scheme, in whatever discipline you choose, after completing your initial two foundation years), she was still more junior than any registrar or consultant.

Farah was a lovely person – kind, caring, funny and supportive. To be frank, I even used to wonder sometimes why she wanted to be a surgeon at all (a thought that turned out to be oddly prescient just a few short years later, when I discovered she had ultimately quit her surgical training to become a Radiologist instead). She was also very headstrong and, for want of a better phrase, refused to take any crap from anyone. This was a personality trait I actually really admired in Farah. Unfortunately, it also made her a lot of enemies amongst the ranks of the Vascular registrars and consultants. One of the consultants she especially managed to rub up the wrong way was Mr Chin – but more on that later...

So why did so many of the more senior Vascular surgeons dislike Farah, especially when she was also more than capable at her job? I soon arrived at the disheartening conclusion that the answer was male bravado, pure and simple. At that time, there were only three female doctors working in that Vascular department: fellow FY1 Rebecca, stern Irish consultant Ms Hartigan, and Farah (Cindy 'I've been the ward bitch already' hadn't yet joined us). As a result, the entire department felt very much like a man's domain, with most of the male surgeons holding the thinly veiled view that their (few) female colleagues should, essentially, keep their place. And when it became clear that Farah – *gasp* – had a mind of her own, and was more than prepared to stick up for herself if needs be, many of her male colleagues turned on her.

Halfway into my Vascular rotation, Farah moved to a different, somewhat smaller, hospital (not for any ominous reason – it just so happened the core surgical trainees were on rotations that were two months out of step with those of the FY1 doctors). The smaller hospitals in our locality sometimes needed to refer complex vascular patients to us, as we were, if you can believe it, a specialist vascular centre for the region.

I was sat on the ward with Mr Prabath one day, a few weeks after Farah had left, when his work mobile began ringing. Mr Prabath was on call that day, which meant it was his responsibility to carry the work phone and field calls from other healthcare professionals who wanted to refer surgical patients to us. Only hearing Mr Prabath's (invariably wholly unenthusiastic) end of these conversations was always a fascinating experience. Without question, my favourite exchange had been the following conversation between Mr Prabath and a GP who was worried that his patient may have frostbite:

[*Loud sigh*] "So, you're saying that the patient's toes are black? Look, are you sure it's not just dirt?"

On this occasion, the person ringing Mr Prabath about a possible admission just happened to be Farah. Mr Prabath, like most of his fellow registrars and consultants, had never professed to be Farah's biggest fan. However, whenever I had seen them together, he had been nothing but respectful and

58

professional, and I had deduced from this that maybe, just maybe, he was able to rise above the petty snobbery of his surgical colleagues.

I was wrong.

When he picked up the phone and realised it was Farah on the other end of the line, what followed (though I didn't realise it at first) was a veritable masterclass in how to be two-faced.

After dutifully listening to Farah relay the patient's history, he agreed to accept the patient as a hospital transfer (to be transported across later that afternoon), before proceeding to ask Farah how she was getting on at her new hospital. Some brief chitchat followed, before Mr Prabath ended the call by cheerfully telling Farah how lovely it had been to speak to her, and how he really hoped they'd be able to catch up properly soon.

As soon as he ended the call, his expression immediately changed to one of annoyance, before I heard him gruffly mutter under his breath, "Damn woman never shuts up."

Never straying far from the 'party line', the boy was back in town.

TAKING IT ON THE CHIN

I mentioned earlier that Farah had a particularly tempestuous relationship with Mr Chin, one of the Vascular consultants. Mr Chin was, to put it mildly, a bit of an oddity. Like most of the consultants in that department, he wasn't exactly the cuddliest of individuals, a fact that also stretched to some of his personal habits. He had two especially off-putting behaviours, which would quickly become apparent to anyone unfortunate enough to spend any appreciable length of time in the man's company: snorting loudly whenever his nose felt blocked and, worse still, talking with his mouth full whenever he ate. What most certainly didn't help the latter was the fact his teeth were quite crooked, meaning food often got stuck between them. It didn't exactly make for a pretty sight.

His sense of humour also left a lot to be desired. I will never forget the following bizarre exchange between myself and Mr Chin (occurring, I should point out, in the company of three other senior surgeons), which still baffles me to this day:

"You know, Ahmed, you're looking a little pale," Mr Chin randomly opined one day, completely out of the blue.

"I'm fine, Mr Chin," I replied, adding, "Perhaps I just need to get out more – get a bit more sun."

"Tell me," Mr Chin went on, "do you have any relatives who live in Wales?"

Having absolutely no idea where exactly this peculiar and seemingly disjointed exchange was heading, I replied, "Erm, well, I do actually have an aunt and uncle who live in Cardiff, Mr Chin."

"Ah," Mr Chin mused, "that explains why you're so pale, then – must be all that sheep-shagging."

The other surgeons present all laughed, albeit a little hesitantly. I let out a small, forced chuckle (frankly, it was all I could think to do in that moment) before Mr Chin suddenly lost all interest in his conversation with me and resumed chatting with the other surgeons. It's fair to say that the sheep-shagging exchange (now *there's* a sentence I never thought I'd ever write) neatly sums up Mr Chin's unique sense of humour: aiming for funny, but invariably missing the mark and landing squarely on the bizarre.

When I first knew Mr Chin, he'd given the impression of being pretty unflappable; someone who wasn't really bothered by anyone or anything. Part of this stemmed from a moment early on in my Vascular rotation when I was doing some audit work in the secretaries' office one Friday afternoon. For Mr Chin, Friday afternoon was, ostensibly, his half-day paperwork session. However, I soon discovered that the Vascular surgeons at our hospital received so many patient complaints (having read this far into Part II of this book you're probably beginning to build up a reasonable picture as to why) that the consultants had begun informally referring to these administrative half-days as their 'complaints sessions'. Not long after my arrival that particular Friday afternoon, Mr Chin emerged from his office, a beaming smile on his face. He turned to his secretary, and cheerfully remarked, "Fantastic! I've only had three

61

complaints this week!" In that moment, I silently dreaded to think what a bad week for Mr Chin looked like.

However, such moments aside, I quickly found out that Mr Chin was anything but unflappable. Indeed, it transpired that he had a particular reputation for seeming nice on the surface, but also being capable of turning on you very quickly, and severely, if you did something that displeased him. Indeed, a particular expression was even coined for those unlucky enough to be on the receiving end of one of Mr Chin's outbursts: "Damn – you just got *chinned*."

As I alluded to before, one person who was unfortunate enough to end up getting 'chinned' repeatedly was the long-suffering Farah. Indeed, such was the intensity of Mr Chin's dislike for Farah that it failed to diminish even after she moved hospital.

I mentioned earlier that, in her new placement, Farah would occasionally have to refer patients to us. I remember my FY1 colleague, Marcus, relaying a story to me about one such occasion with genuine shock. On the day in question, one of the registrars was going through that afternoon's list of new patient admissions with Mr Chin, when he happened to highlight the fact that one of them (Mr Sellers) was a hospital transfer patient who had been referred in by Farah. Immediately, Mr Chin flew into a rage.

"Wait – so the patient was referred in by *that* incompetent imbecile? [*Loud sigh*] Look, as soon as Mr Sellers gets here, I want you to begin from scratch – start by taking the entire history again. I'm *not* going to trust a single word that stupid woman might have said to you over the phone!"

So why, you may ask, did Mr Chin dislike Farah so

intensely? Well, I suspect the answer may at least partly be rooted in an unfortunate incident that took place in theatre some months earlier – one that turned out to be one of the unexpected highlights of my entire four months in vascular surgery. To give proper context to this story, I should explain that Mr Chin originally hailed from Beijing, and Farah's family from Iran.

Mr Chin and Farah were washing their hands (aka getting scrubbed) in theatre, preparing to operate on a patient. Mr Chin was, as you've already discovered, never one to shy away from an inappropriate joke or two, and it just so happened that there had been a terrorist bombing in Iran just two days earlier.

Smirking, Mr Chin turned to Farah and said, "I hear from the news that *your boys* have been up to no good recently. Tsk tsk."

Farah was visibly taken aback, but without missing a beat, calmly retorted, "Yes, that's true. But haven't you heard, Mr Chin? These days, all the world's best terrorists come from China."

To say that Mr Chin was thoroughly unamused by Farah's quip would be a gross understatement. But for me personally, leaving aside the undeniably wrong and immature race-baiting, I couldn't help but feel a swell of respect for Farah in that moment as she refused to simply 'keep her place', lie down and take her boss' insensitive comments. In other words, damn – *he* just got chinned.

I AM THE WALRUS

Next up in the Vascular rogues' gallery was the department's very own (and please pardon the overbearing stench of sarcasm) ray of sunshine, Mr Jones. Bald, overweight, and sporting a distinctive walrus moustache, Mr Jones was undoubtedly one of the gruffest individuals you could ever hope (or not) to meet. He was foul-mouthed, utterly uncompromising, and had a manner that instantly told you that he was *not* someone you wanted to piss off; indeed, there was an unmistakeable fire perpetually visible behind his eyes, which his oval glasses only seemed to magnify.

Mr Jones was actually the first Vascular consultant I met when I started the job, and his demeanour at that initial meeting was, sadly, but the first sign of the rough ride that was to follow over the next four months. Our departmental 'induction' (and I do use that term loosely) was essentially a five minute lecture in how not to rub him or any of the other consultants up the wrong way. Most memorable was this choice gem:

"And look, I personally don't give a fuck if you leave the hospital early one day, so long as you get all your work done [note: this never *once* happened]. But as far as I'm concerned, if I bleep you, and *someone* doesn't pick up, then you should be fucking sacked."

So, as you've probably gathered, Mr Jones was not a man

who minced his words. He liked things to be done a particular way – his way – and if they weren't, then you were going to get a bollocking, pure and simple. Indeed, I remember one morning when he came onto the ward just prior to one of his (rare) ward rounds, and first proceeded to cast his eye over the white board behind the doctors' desk (this listed the names of all the ward's patients, beside which were the initials of each individual's named consultant). Suddenly, he spotted something on the board that clearly met with his disapproval, as the fire behind his eyes suddenly intensified tenfold.

"The lady in bed six!" he barked at me. "She is *not* my fucking patient. Rub my initials off from next to her name, and do it now. If something goes off with her, then I am *not* going to take fucking responsibility for it."

I soon discovered that not wanting to take responsibility for things was a bit of a recurring theme when it came to Mr Jones. Twice a week, the Vascular department would hold a multidisciplinary team (MDT) meeting, attended by consultants, registrars, interventional Radiologists (who were there to help interpret patients' angiograms – a type of x-ray used to image blood vessels), and junior doctors. At these meetings, complex patients would be discussed, and a consensus decision then reached as to how best to proceed with their management. Invariably, Mr Jones's sole contributions to these meetings would always be the same: whatever the patient's story and clinical background, as soon as he saw their angiogram pictures on the projector screen, he'd gruffly opine from the back of the room, "I wouldn't go anywhere near that – you'll just bugger up their arteries."

Sadly, Mr Jones's attitude towards patients was no less

blunt than that towards his colleagues. I remember an (understandably horrified) fellow junior doctor recounting the story of when they'd once accompanied Mr Jones as he'd reviewed a patient with leg pain. The patient had been admitted to the Surgical Assessment Unit (SAU) during Mr Jones's on call.

"So," Mr Jones began somewhat apathetically, "when did this pain start?"

The patient then proceeded to describe his pain in great detail: its exact location, how severe it was, and the other symptoms which accompanied it. Mid-flow, Mr Jones suddenly cut him off abruptly.

"Stop. Shut the fuck up. That is *not* what I asked you. When did the pain first start?"

My colleague, I suspect, was left even more shocked by Mr Jones's words than the patient. Forget complaints; how such incidents failed to generate column inches in a newspaper remains a genuine mystery to me. I'd be lying if I said I didn't sometimes wish that certain patients came with a mute button, but telling them to *shut the fuck up*... I mean, really?

At the start of my time in vascular surgery, I had wondered if Mr Jones's tetchy demeanour was simply a façade he put on at work – another example of the 'dick swinging' culture so prevalent within that department. I soon discovered, however, that Mr Jones would behave in pretty much exactly the same manner outside of work too.

Once every few weeks, the registrars and junior doctors would all get together on a Thursday night after work at a bar downtown and invariably stay out far too late, and occasionally drink far too much. I'd like to think that the registrars never actually turned up hungover for their Friday morning theatre lists though, worryingly, I have my doubts.

Occasionally, the consultants would join us on these nights out, Mr Jones included. To be honest, I was never quite sure why he did, since he seemed just as grumpy and miserable outside of work as he did at the hospital. During one work night out, my junior doctor colleague, Marcus, even offered Mr Jones a glass of whiskey he'd just bought for him at the bar, only for the latter to bark, "No! Get that fucking disgusting drink away from me!"

So no, tact and diplomacy were most definitely not amongst Mr Jones's strong suits. I even recall a cringe-worthy ward round he led in which he curtly explained to a lady on SAU (who'd come in with abdominal pain) why he thought her pain had a gynaecological rather than a surgical cause (a classic example of yet another sadly true-to-life surgical cliché: *always* first assume that your female patient's tummy pain must be gynaecological in origin, rather than anything you should be dealing with yourself). When the befuddled-looking patient then asked Mr Jones (who had already turned to walk away) what the term gynaecological meant, a look of almost revulsion appeared across his face, as though he had suddenly just stepped in a large cow pat. "Oh, you know – *women's bits.*"

You'd never guess that a smooth talker like Mr Jones was married, would you?

As I mentioned earlier, surgeons often get a bad reputation for their perceived lack of empathy and compassion towards patients, a sentiment that – as you've probably already gathered – experience has forced me to agree is sadly sometimes true. No single incident sums this up as well as one involving Mr Jones and a green needle...

During one particular on call on SAU, I clerked in Mr Argyll, a pleasant diabetic gentleman who had been referred in by his GP with a rather nasty-looking ulcer over the sole of his right foot. This is sadly a common complication in patients with poorly controlled diabetes. Compounding matters is the fact that persistently high blood sugar levels can also lead to nerve damage, resulting in a loss of sensation in a diabetic patient's foot.

On returning to the doctors' desk from the patient's bedside, I noticed that Mr Jones was hovering somewhat impatiently (he happened to be the consultant on call that day).

"So, what have you got for me?" Mr Jones asked in his characteristically gruff tone of voice.

I proceeded to relay Mr Argyll's history to a rather disinterested-looking Mr Jones. Once I had finished my summary, Mr Jones curtly asked me to fetch him a green needle from the store cupboard, and then join him by the patient's bedside. Without another word, he then strolled off in the direction of Mr Argyll's bed.

A green needle? I was genuinely puzzled. What on earth did Mr Jones want one of those for? Though I knew that it made absolutely no clinical sense, I concluded that Mr Jones must have been planning to drain the patient's ulcer. Why else would he need the needle? I promptly picked up a green needle from the store cupboard, along with a ten millilitre syringe and a few gauze swabs, before rejoining Mr Jones at Mr Argyll's bedside.

As he took an unimpressed look at the non-needle

equipment I had brought him, Mr Jones dismissively growled, "No, I don't need any of that gubbins!"

Then, with one swift motion, Mr Jones picked up the green needle, unsheathed it from its protective plastic covering and, without a word of warning, or a moment's hesitation, suddenly stuck the needle, full force, into Mr Argyll's foot ulcer.

I could feel all the air suddenly leave my lungs. Was this man *insane*?

"Did that hurt?" Mr Jones asked the patient matter-of-factly.

To my immense and lasting relief, Mr Argyll shook his head, and my heart beat again.

If I didn't know it before, then I most definitely knew it in that moment. The rumours had been true: these Vascular consultants really *were* psychotic.

MACHO MACHO MAN

As I reflect back on my time in vascular surgery, it's genuinely difficult to pick a personal 'least favourite' amongst all the consultants, but a worthy contender would most definitely be the head of department, Mr Agrawal. He was, by all accounts, the very embodiment of someone with small man syndrome; his muscular physique was somewhat at odds with his diminutive height, a fact that gave him a chip on his shoulder the size of a horse. He also had an accent that entirely defied explanation. Though his family were originally from Sri Lanka, and he had trained in Northern Ireland, he somehow permanently sounded like he was doing a poor imitation of someone from Boston, Massachusetts. This gave his diction some very specific, and peculiar, quirks. For instance, he would characteristically drag out the final syllable of any word ending with an 'ah' or 'ar' sound so that it became a bizarrely elongated 'errr'– a fact I discovered, to my amusement, when I curiously heard him refer to one of our patients (whose first name was Lisa) as "Lees-errrrr." I soon found that I could imitate Mr Agrawal with a fair degree of accuracy, to the amusement of my colleagues. Hell, I even once sang karaoke at a friend's house party *as* Mr Agrawal (the song was *Common People* by Pulp, if you're curious). Before long though, I did begin to regret having honed this particular impression when certain registrars and even consultants got wind of it and, to my embarrassment, would even ask me to repeat it in front of them like some kind of party trick. My fear was that the impression would eventually get back to Mr Agrawal (thankfully, as far as I know, it never did), someone who most emphatically did *not* have a sense of humour when it came to such things.

At his core, I saw Mr Agrawal as someone who just wanted to be loved by everyone. I vividly remember the talk he gave us on vascular surgery during the FY1 whole-year group induction the day before that very first Black Wednesday. While most of that day's speakers had come dressed to the nines in smart suits and ties, and lectured to us with the aid of dry PowerPoint presentations, Mr Agrawal strolled into the seminar room casual as anything, wearing lightly ripped jeans and a shirt with its sleeves rolled up well past his elbows. He immediately picked up one of the chairs, spun it around so that its back was towards his audience, set it down close to the front row, and sat facing the crowd, before proceeding to nonchalantly ask, "So, what do you guys wanna know about vascular surgery?"

Sure, he seemed pleasant enough (at least, he did back then), but it was also achingly obvious to all of us just how hard he was trying to be 'one of the gang'; hell, all he would've needed to complete the illusion was a backwards-facing baseball cap and a jacket emblazoned with the words *Cool Dude*. However, while Mr Agrawal may have looked like he wanted to be everybody's friend on the surface, it soon transpired (once I'd started my surgical rotation) that he had a darker side lurking beneath that seemingly affable exterior.

Once you began working alongside him, some things

quickly became apparent about Mr Agrawal. For instance, he generally treated his female juniors better than his male ones, principally because he had an unapologetic eye for the ladies. As an example, I remember one particular day when Mr Agrawal came onto the ward, looking to assign some jobs to the FY1s. I happened to be on the ward at the time with my FY1 colleague, Rebecca.

"Rebecc-errrrr." Mr Agrawal beamed at her, an unmistakeable twinkle in his eye. "I have a job for you of the utmost importance," he said in a mock-serious tone. "Your mission, should you choose to accept it, is to take bloods from the lady in bed eight before we take her down to theatre. Do you think you can do that for me?" When she cheerfully agreed to his request, he winked at her, jovially declaring, "That's my girl!" As soon as Rebecca had set off towards bed eight, he turned to me, the smile instantly disappearing from his face. "Ahmed," he said dourly, "there's a stack of discharge summaries that need doing on the Day Admissions Unit – the ward sister has been getting on my back about them. Go now, please."

Another fact we all soon learned was that Mr Agrawal had a definite mean streak; stories of him going into a rage and yelling venomously in theatre at registrars who had displeased him were not uncommon (and were also sadly par for the course in that particular department). What I didn't discover until a fair while later, however, was that if his machismo and sense of male pride were in any way threatened, Mr Agrawal could become childishly petty, and incredibly vicious. Sadly, it was my fellow Vascular FY1 and friend, Luke, who most harshly bore the brunt of Mr Agrawal's wrath.

Everybody loved Luke. A short man with a big heart, Luke was a proper lads' lad, in a way that Mr Agrawal could (and presumably did) only dream of. It must be said that Luke was not always necessarily the sharpest tool in the surgical box. One particular incident immediately springs to mind in that regard, involving a gentleman who had had, somewhat unusually, a cancerous growth surgically removed from his scalp. He was recuperating on the ward post-op, with a large, white circular dressing adorning the top of his head. As the registrar leading our ward round began speaking to the patient, Luke (who'd never met the gentleman before) quickly went off to retrieve his notes from the trolley. By the time he re-emerged inside the patient's cubicle, notes in hand (and flanked by an eager fourth year medical student), he'd missed the entirety of the initial discussion between the patient and the registrar. While Luke was flicking to the right page in the gentleman's records, the medical student leant in and whispered:

"Luke, why is the patient wearing that on his head?"

Luke looked quizzically at the patient, then turned back to the student and replied with complete sincerity, "I think he must be Jewish."

And no, we never let him live that one down. Indeed, I imagine that the nurses on the surgical wards must have been thoroughly bemused as to why some of the FY1s suddenly began greeting Luke for weeks afterwards with a tongue-in-cheek, "Shalom."

The odd case of mistaken religious identity aside, Luke did, as I mentioned, have a heart of gold, and was incredibly well-liked. A rugby player, and a self-proclaimed budding surgeon, he also quickly developed a reputation for the sheer quantity of alcohol he could put away on a night out. I actually discovered this the first time I met Luke (during a junior doctors' night out), when he quickly became so plastered that he simply couldn't remember my name. At around 2:00 a.m. that morning, having just asked me (for what must have been the fourth time) what my name was, he suddenly cut me off before I could reply, placed a hand on my shoulder, and drunkenly proclaimed, "You know what? I'm just not gonna remember it, am I? Tell you what, I'm just gonna call you Prince." And so it was that, from that day onwards, despite bearing less than a passing resemblance to the late singer (and that's if I'm being generous), I would come to be known as Prince by many of my FY1 colleagues, some of whom still call me it to this day. I definitely got off lightly, though. You see, Luke also developed a reputation for getting drunk and then – ahem – proceeding to show off 'Luke junior' to all those in attendance. I guess I was fortunate in that I never had to meet him myself.

With his gregarious, friendly nature, Luke's popularity extended not just to his fellow FY1s, but equally to medical students, registrars, and even some consultants, all of whom he would more than happily share a pint (or six) with – and maybe even introduce to Luke junior, God help them. Unfortunately for Luke, his exuberant and easy-going personality could very occasionally get him into trouble, which brings us back to Mr Agrawal.

As I mentioned earlier, the junior doctors, registrars and occasionally consultants would sometimes go for a work night out on a Thursday. There was one particular team social that ended up becoming infamous amongst the Vascular team, and which also somewhat soured the tone for all the nights out that followed. Truth be told, I wasn't actually there myself during this particular evening sojourn into the city centre (this was just a few days after my mum had passed away), and so the following story was actually conveyed to me by my colleague, Marcus, who ended up bearing witness to a bizarre incident involving Luke and Mr Agrawal.

In short, to the surprise of no one, Luke ended up drinking far too much. Mr Agrawal became determined to keep up with him, and before long the two men were both completely hammered. Discovering, to his dismay, that he was simply unable to out-drink Luke (which to be fair was always going to be a losing battle from the start), but unwilling to be outplayed by an FY1 twenty-five years his junior, Mr Agrawal decided, as you do, to challenge Luke to a one-armed push-up contest. Luke, also not one to be outdone, eagerly agreed. Without a moment's hesitation, Luke – in a surprising and impressive display of dexterity for someone with such a large quantity of alcohol coursing through their veins – immediately launched into a series of one-armed push-ups, carried out with enthusiastic vigour. Mr Agrawal, on the other hand, struggled to complete even a scant few push-ups before (in Marcus's words) "collapsing to the floor in a pathetic, wheezy heap." On witnessing his easy victory Luke, still fuelled by significant amounts of Jägermeister and vodka, immediately leaped to his feet and, in a shining example of the very opposite of magnanimity in victory, began taunting the still floored Mr Agrawal with a triumphant: "Yes! Yes! Los-er! Looos-errr!"

It was an incident none of the team would soon forget, not least of which Mr Agrawal. But the ego-bruised consultant didn't take his revenge straight away. No, that actually happened a week later, with Mr Agrawal's unlikely weapon of choice turning out to be something that would otherwise seem entirely innocuous: the theatre list running order.

Forget taking bloods and writing endless hospital discharge summaries – by far the single most banal of all a surgical FY1's daily responsibilities was filling out the theatre list running order, i.e. the specific order in which elective operations were scheduled to take place the following day. Now, the consultants would each keep a copy of their own theatre list in their secretary's diary, with the operations invariably having already been put into the consultant's desired running order (based on factors such as each patient's medical history, or the availability of particular surgical equipment). Our job as Vascular FY1s (a chore which extended to other surgical specialties as well) was to take it in turns to head down each morning to the Vascular secretaries' office (which was housed in a Portakabin a ten minute walk away from the main hospital building), copy down the next day's theatre list running order from the relevant secretary's diary onto a separate piece of paper, then head back to the main hospital building, walk to theatres, and hand said piece of paper in at the reception desk. This all had to be done before midday in order to give theatre staff the opportunity to adequately prepare for the following day's theatre list.

What, precisely, the exact point was of this peculiar little ritual still baffles me to this day. Why couldn't the consultants just write down the running order at the theatre reception desk, as opposed to in their secretary's diary? Alternatively, why couldn't the secretaries simply ring up theatres themselves and relay the next day's running order verbally over the phone? And why had this bizarre practice seemingly never before been questioned or (heaven forbid) clearly explained, even after several years, with scores of obliging FY1s having dutifully carried it out? These were just three questions to which I never came up with satisfactory answers. Sure, this arguably pointless daily chore was hardly mentally taxing, but it did take a good thirty minute chunk out of an FY1's already extremely packed day, and was also always potentially open to error. Though thankfully it didn't happen very often, FY1s would occasionally make a mistake while transcribing the running order from one piece of paper to another and, if they did, then the consultant carrying out said theatre list would almost certainly make their displeasure known to them in their typically vocal, profanity-laden way.

On the Wednesday following 'push-up gate', it happened to be Luke's turn to transcribe the following day's theatre list running order, which just so happened to be Mr Agrawal's list. Just as he had done several times before, Luke dutifully copied the list down from Mr Agrawal's secretary's diary, and handed it in at theatre reception before midday. His menial task done, Luke went back to his other ward duties and thought no more about it.

The next day, we were halfway through the morning, registrar-led ward round when, from inside a patient cubicle at the very end of the ward, we suddenly heard a booming, furious-sounding voice emanating from the doctors' desk some distance away – the inimitable voice of Mr Agrawal.

"Luke! Luke Jameson! Get your sorry self over here ... NOW!"

Visibly alarmed, Luke handed me the set of patient notes

in which he'd been writing, and hastily walked over to the doctors' desk. As myself, my colleague Marcus and our registrar remained in the cubicle (attempting to maintain some sense of professionalism in front of the now bewildered-looking patient), Mr Agrawal's venomous screaming could clearly be heard by everyone from one end of the ward to the other – not to mention, I would imagine, those in the neighbouring ward as well.

"You screwed up big time, Luke! You wrote out today's theatre list, didn't you? You put Mrs Palmer second in the running order when I'd *specifically* put her first! Are you completely fucking stupid?! Mrs Palmer is a type 1 diabetic. Like I've told you all a *thousand* times, patients on insulin always need to be done first on the operating list! Now we're going to have to postpone her operation, and that's on *you*! Copying down the theatre list isn't exactly hard, is it? And yet somehow you've managed to fuck it up! You are, without doubt, the most incompetent junior who's ever worked for me!!"

Though it was virtually impossible to hear anything above the din of Mr Agrawal's shouting, one could just about make out a meek-sounding Luke within the melee trying to justify himself in a small, apologetic tone of voice. Mr Agrawal, of course, was having none of it and soon stormed off the ward in a huff, just as quickly as he'd bulldozed onto it minutes earlier.

When the dust had settled, and the rest of us had returned to the doctors' desk, the sight that greeted us was a rather stunned-looking Luke, staring off into the distance, his expression a mixture of embarrassment, guilt and shock, a world away from the easy-going man I'd come to know. Taking a look around, it also quickly became apparent just how many people had witnessed what had just happened (either visibly, audibly, or both): nurses, healthcare assistants and, worst of all, what must have been most if not all of the ward's patients. You could tell that everyone was a little taken aback, and at first no one quite knew what to say.

All of us were furious on Luke's behalf. Not only was Mr Agrawal's angry tirade rude, demeaning, and hugely unprofessional, it also flagrantly breached poor Mrs Palmer's confidentiality to anyone within earshot. Luke himself was more confused than anything; how, he thought, could he have made such a foolish error? His confusion was only matched by his guilt. He felt terrible that Mrs Palmer's operation had had to be postponed, seemingly because of him; so terrible that he became determined to find out just what had gone wrong. And here's the rub: it transpired that, seemingly, the only thing Luke had perhaps done wrong was to show up Mr Agrawal in a drunken one-armed push-up contest.

When Luke returned to the secretaries' office to investigate what had happened, he rechecked the theatre list running order that Mr Agrawal had written in his secretary's diary, noting that Mrs Palmer was indeed first on the operating list. Later, when he went to theatre reception, he asked them to recheck the list he had handed in, only to discover Mrs Palmer was, in fact, first on *that* list too.

All that we could surmise was that either someone in theatres had screwed up on the day and bumped Mrs Palmer to second in the running order by mistake ... or else no one had messed up at all, and the whole sorry 'misunderstanding' had been concocted by Mr Agrawal in a petty attempt to embarrass

Luke in front of his patients, his peers and his seniors. For Mrs Palmer's sake, I very much hope that her operation being postponed really was just down to an innocent mistake – but I sadly very much have my doubts. I think Luke did too, which is why he chose not to present his 'evidence' to Mr Agrawal, electing instead to simply keep his distance from the man for the rest of the rotation. To my mind, Luke never received an apology over the incident, which certainly left a bitter taste in my mouth (let alone his), and only served as yet another reminder of the toxic environment in which I was working.

I mentioned earlier that Luke was a budding surgeon when I first met him. I don't think it's entirely coincidental that he soon changed his mind and decided to become an anaesthetist instead. I don't imagine that Luke was especially sad to see the back of his four months in vascular surgery – and neither, as you can no doubt tell, was I.

PART III

OBSTETRICS & GYNAECOLOGY

AHMED AND THE DRAGON

Thursday AM – Theatre, MOB.

This is what my timetable read for my first proper day in Obstetrics & Gynaecology (aka Obs & Gynae, or simply O&G), following our whistle-stop departmental induction the previous day. MOB was the acronym for one of the O&G consultants and the person who would be my clinical supervisor for the next four months: Ms Molly O'Brien.

A few days before starting in O&G, I had briefly met Peter, a fellow FY1, on labour ward at the end of the day. He was just finishing his O&G rotation, and I was meeting him to collect his (now my) bleep, as I would be taking over his post. I asked him what my new boss, Ms O'Brien, was like.

"She's a little bit scary," he replied matter-of-factly. "She's a bit like Ms Hartigan, actually – Irish, and doesn't take any prisoners."

I had of course just completed a four-month rotation in vascular surgery under the supervision of Ms Hartigan and, although we hadn't exactly got on like a house on fire, I'd certainly come across a lot worse. *Okay, so she's a bit like Ms Hartigan*, I mused to myself. *How bad could she be?* As I've learned time and time again over the years, idly saying – or even thinking – such things is *never* a good idea.

I walked onto the Day Admissions Unit at 8:30 a.m. sharp

on that first Thursday morning, eager to impress. Helpfully, Peter had told me that Ms O'Brien always came to see all the patients on her morning theatre list about half an hour before the list started. After arriving at the unit, pre-printed patient list in hand, I quickly noticed that the curtains had already been drawn around the bay of the first patient on the morning list. After a brief conversation with one of the nurses, I discovered it was Ms O'Brien behind the curtains, and from the muffled sounds of her Irish brogue it was clear she was already halfway through consenting the patient. This meant that even though I had arrived bang on time, she had come in before me – and that essentially meant I was late. Not the most auspicious of starts.

I decided to wait until Ms O'Brien had finished with the patient, reasoning that waltzing in halfway through the surgical consent process would not be the most appropriate way for me to introduce myself for the very first time.

The diminutive figure of Ms O'Brien soon emerged from the patient bay and, once she'd spotted me (even though we'd never met before), instantly seemed to know who I was.

"Ah, you must be Achmed," she said, not bothering to find out whether or not she'd pronounced my name correctly (she hadn't). "So, I've just consented Mrs Ellis for a laparoscopy. Her GP referred her to my clinic last month with a six-month history of pelvic pain. What are the most common gynaecological causes of pelvic pain?"

I froze, suddenly (in my mind, at least) resembling a fox that had just had a light shone in its face. It had been over two years since I had completed my six-week attachment in O&G at medical school and, despite my best efforts, this on-the-spot grilling (a teaching technique, as I mentioned earlier, that I have always loathed) had instantly made all that knowledge mostly inaccessible.

Ms O'Brien had the kind of face that made you suspect she'd secretly been sucking on a lemon for the past twenty years, and the sort of eyes that seemed to bore deeply into your soul. I managed to pass a half-hearted, admittedly less than stellar, answer from my lips. To say that she did not look impressed would be an understatement.

"Well, it's nice to see that you came here prepared," she replied sarcastically.

And that was how it began: my four months under the tutelage of a consultant who, thanks to my endless hours spent complaining about her down the phone, my dad soon came to dub 'The Dragon Lady'.

I very quickly began to loathe Thursday mornings and, to be frank, pretty much everything about Ms O'Brien. I didn't like her attitude with patients; I didn't like the way she would badmouth her colleagues to pretty much all and sundry; and I definitely didn't like the way she treated me. For the entirety of the four months I spent working for her, I consistently felt on edge, in a way I don't think I have before or since. I don't think she actively disliked me – she probably saw her constant put-downs and criticisms as a motivator – but for me, someone who's admittedly always been too sensitive for his own good, they simply left me feeling like a bit of a useless know-nothing, whose mere presence in the job was somehow managing to offend their boss' every sensibility. The irony is, I actually got on pretty well with almost all the other O&G consultants (except perhaps for Mr Parker – but more on him later), and their feedback on my work and clinical performance was almost always positive. So why did Ms O'Brien and I simply not get along? To this day, I'm not entirely certain. With the passing of time I've simply put it down to the chalk and cheese effect – i.e. a fundamental clash of personality types.

To give you more of an idea of just what Ms O'Brien was like, this story, which was relayed to me one day by her registrar, pretty much sums her up perfectly.

A few years before I started there, the O&G department had a Greek locum called Aldous working for them. He was, all things told, a man with a very distinctive look – quite portly, and completely bald.

One summer, Aldous went on annual leave for three weeks – ostensibly, his colleagues all assumed, for a beach holiday in Greece. When he returned, however, it immediately became apparent something was different: he now had a lush headful of hair.

Very quickly, Aldous's hair transplant became the proverbial elephant in the room amongst his colleagues. Tempting though it was, everyone quietly and tacitly agreed that the most diplomatic approach would simply be to avoid all mention of Aldous's new luscious locks.

Coincidentally, Ms O'Brien was herself on holiday during Aldous's hairy (sorry!) first week back at work. On the day of her return, she came up to labour ward at 5:00 p.m. to receive handover for her evening on call shift from none other than Aldous.

And what, you might ask, was the very first thing Ms O'Brien said upon seeing Aldous, in the company of at least half a dozen other doctors and midwives?

"Aldous! What the fuck have you done to your hair?"

You get the idea.

What I always found especially bizarre is that Ms O'Brien was actually very much like Marmite to her patients: they either absolutely adored her, or else they *despised* her. Indeed, whenever I would see patients coming out of Ms O'Brien's consulting room, they would typically be saying one of two very distinct things to whomever had accompanied them:

"Oh, I do like that Ms O'Brien. She just gives it to you straight, and tells it like it is." Or, "You know, I really can't stand that woman. She's bossy, rude, and didn't listen to a word I said!"

One of Ms O'Brien's seemingly favourite phrases (one of many I quickly grew to hate) was something I would hear her say to some of her patients as she consented them for theatre on the morning of their operation. As does sometimes happen with surgical procedures, the patient will occasionally have been seen by someone else in clinic (e.g. one of the registrars, or a different consultant) but then be operated on by Ms O'Brien herself. This could (mostly due to differences in the way that different doctors explain the same thing) result in a patient agreeing to undergo a particular procedure in clinic, and then later becoming confused when seemingly being consented for a slightly different procedure on the day of their operation.

"But I don't understand, Ms O'Brien," some patients would say. "They told me in clinic that I'd be having—"

Ms O'Brien would always interrupt at this point, defiantly snarling, "They? Who's *they*? *I'm* the they!"

This Marmite reaction extended to Ms O'Brien's consultant colleagues and juniors as well. To both my consternation and utter bafflement, many of those she worked with absolutely loved her, and would go on at length about how lovely and supportive Molly was (only those who liked her ever referred to her by her first name). Anna, one of the medical students in O&G, even told me that Ms O'Brien had once personally paid for both Anna and a group of other students to fly out to Rome for a Gynaecology conference, like she was some kind of Mother Teresa for women's health.

Honestly, whenever I would hear such stories I almost questioned whether or not they were actually talking about the same person. Ms O'Brien? Lovely and supportive? Were they joking? Scratch that – were they *high*?

I mentioned the film *Zoolander* a little earlier in this book. For those of you who haven't seen it, there's a moment towards the end of the film when Will Ferrell's character, Jacobim Mugatu, angrily rants at the audience at a fashion show, desperately trying to convince them that the hero, hapless buffoon Derek Zoolander, actually only has one modelling 'look', despite everyone constantly praising him for his versatility.

'The man has one look, for Christ's sake! [...] Doesn't anyone notice this?! I feel like I'm taking crazy pills!'

Yes, for four unhappy months, I felt very much like Jacobim Mugatu, railing against a clearly ridiculous character, only to frequently be met with a series of blank stares. Honestly, the first time I met a colleague who admitted to disliking Ms O'Brien as much as I did, I wanted to hug them; finally, here was proof that I wasn't crazy, the cathartic validation I'd so desperately been looking for.

The oft heard references to Ms O'Brien's 'supportive

nature' left me particularly mystified. I certainly never felt that, as my boss, she ever really had my back, a feeling best illustrated by an incident that occurred about halfway through my rotation.

Each Wednesday, the junior doctors would be given their timetable for the following week. One of the great things about O&G was its great variety: theatre, labour ward, antenatal clinics, Gynae clinics, ward rounds, on call commitments and more would all typically feature on the timetable each week, which certainly helped to keep things from ever becoming routine or monotonous (indeed, I think that variety is a big part of why I now love being a GP). Next to each clinic listed on the timetable, it would tell you exactly who was going to be in clinic with you (e.g. which consultant and/or registrar); typically, there would be two or three clinicians allocated to each clinic. As I picked up my latest timetable one Wednesday, however, I couldn't help but notice that it was only myself who'd been assigned to do Ms O'Brien's Gynae clinic the following Wednesday morning, as both Ms O'Brien and her registrar were on leave that week.

Now, being assigned to Ms O'Brien's clinic while the sourpuss herself was absent was usually a cause for quiet celebration, but not this time. Here I was, a first year junior doctor, with a grand total of eight weeks of O&G experience, and I was being asked to run Ms O'Brien's Gynae clinic all by myself, without any kind of senior support. Surely this was a mistake?

When I enquired about this seeming error to the (non-clinical) rota co-ordinator, she flatly and disinterestedly told me to take up my concerns with Ms O'Brien. Oh joy. And so it was that I bit the bullet, knocked on the door of The Dragon Lady's office, and explained my predicament to her. And what was her helpful and supportive response?

"Look, Achmed [no, she still couldn't pronounce my name properly, and no, she never did] – you've been doing this job for eight weeks now, and so I expect you to be able to manage being in clinic on your own." In other words, the clinic arrangements for the following week stood, and logic (not to mention patient care) be damned. I was genuinely stunned, not to mention wholly overwhelmed at the prospect of the upcoming clinic, but what more could I do?

I think it was during that Wednesday morning clinic, where I was indeed the only doctor present, that my resentment of Ms O'Brien probably peaked. Yes, they had reduced the number of patients booked into the clinic, and the rota co-ordinator had attempted to appease me by also assigning an advanced nurse practitioner (ANP) to join me in clinic, but such measures failed to address the inherent absurdity of the frankly unsafe position in which I found myself. In short, I felt uncomfortably out of my depth and, in fairness, I'm pretty sure even the most confident of FY1s would have too in that situation. This was no more evident than with my very first patient that day, an incredibly complex lady whose case was so tricky to manage that fellow consultant Mr Parker had actually referred her to Ms O'Brien for a second opinion. So, as the patient herself no doubt also thought, if a consultant had been stumped for ideas, what in the hell was *I* going to add to this lady's clinical management? As I made my profuse apologies to the patient – and promised to personally speak with Ms O'Brien about this lady's care upon the former's return – the disappointed, slightly resentful look on her face really hit hard. She felt like we'd wasted her time, and it was hard to argue with that assessment. I somehow managed to limp my way through the rest of that morning's clinic without too much drama, but I never let go of the anger I felt towards Ms O'Brien for having put me in that situation in the first place.

The more time went on, the worse things seemed to get between myself and Ms O'Brien, to the point where I very quickly began to dread having to pick up the following week's timetable each Wednesday. As soon as I looked down and saw that I'd been assigned to one of Ms O'Brien's clinics or theatre lists, my heart would sink just that little bit deeper. Conversely, discovering that The Dragon Lady was on leave the following week made me feel like a kid on Christmas morning (provided said kid wasn't then forced to do an outpatient clinic solo).

As the weeks and months passed, Ms O'Brien would find ever more inventive ways to scornfully deride my behaviour whenever we were together. For some reason, picking on me was something Ms O'Brien seemed to especially enjoy doing whenever medical students were present. Personally, I think she enjoyed having an audience for her mocking critique.

"Perhaps *you'd* care to tell our student, Achmed," Ms O'Brien asked me during one of her Thursday morning theatre lists, "exactly how many beds we have on labour ward?"

My mind went blank, a frustratingly frequent occurrence in The Dragon Lady's company. The answer was something in the forties, but I couldn't quite remember the precise number.

"I'm not exactly sure, Ms O'Brien," I replied, as my predominant focus remained on ensuring I was still holding the surgical retractor in the very particular way Ms O'Brien had insisted upon. "But I think it might be—"

"Well," she said sarcastically, cutting me off mid-sentence, "well done for taking an active interest in what goes on in our department."

I felt like screaming. I'm also not quite sure who looked more embarrassed – me or the student.

The nadir of this ritual humiliation came at a work social gathering which took place towards the end of my rotation. It was held at a nearby restaurant for one of the registrars, Ayisha, who was shortly going on maternity leave. To be honest, I didn't really want to go at all. The idea of having to spend even a minute in Ms O'Brien's company outside of work was about as enviable as having my fingernails pulled out, but I felt it would've been antisocial of me not to show my face.

The party initially seemed harmless enough (Ayisha's gushing toast to the 'motherly' Ms O'Brien aside – urgh), and I was fortunate enough not to have to speak to The Dragon Lady at all for around the first half hour or so. Inevitably though, she and I did end up having a conversation, flanked by a junior doctor colleague, one of the registrars, and even Ms O'Brien's surprisingly softly-spoken partner.

"You know, I was speaking to Mr Khan [one of the other O&G consultants] earlier, and he told me how impressed he was by your knowledge and work ethic," Ms O'Brien remarked.

A compliment? From The Dragon Lady? Was I hearing things? This had to be too good to be true, surely?

Of course, it was.

"So I told Mr Khan that must be because I've taught you everything I know – because when you joined the department, I thought you were *crap*."

As she laughed mirthlessly, a sea of otherwise awkward-looking faces surrounded me – and I silently prayed for the ground to swallow me up whole.

I'll also never forget one of the very last times I ever saw Ms O'Brien. It was, ironically, just outside the Day Admissions Unit where we'd had that very first inauspicious meeting four months earlier. I was timetabled to be in theatre with her that morning, and knew that, as per usual, she would want to see all the patients on her surgical list from 8:30 a.m. onwards. However, I found myself in a slight quandary on that particular morning. You see, on the previous afternoon I had assisted Mr Khan with his theatre list and, as the FY1, it was my responsibility to review any such post-op patients (whose surgeries you had assisted with) the following morning, with a view to discharging them home if possible. So I wondered, which group of patients should I see first: Mr Khan's post-op ones from the day before, or Ms O'Brien's pre-op ones on the list for that morning?

On balance, I reasoned I would be best off coming into work early, and seeing/discharging Mr Khan's patients first, before proceeding to the Day Admissions Unit and joining Ms O'Brien, which is exactly what I did. What I hadn't anticipated, however, was my own mini-ward round of Mr Khan's patients taking slightly longer than expected, the result of which was that I ended up finishing at 8:40 a.m.

As I hurriedly rushed down the corridor towards the Day Admissions Unit, my heart sank as I saw both Ms O'Brien and her registrar emerging from the unit. As soon as she spotted me, her naturally sour face scrunched into an even deeper scowl – and it was quickly made clear, in no uncertain terms, that I'd made a bad call.

"What the hell do you think you're playing at, Achmed?!", she shrieked at me. "I've just finished seeing the first two patients on this morning's list, and where were you? Fucking AWOL, that's where!"

As I tried to apologetically explain to Ms O'Brien that I had been seeing Mr Khan's patients, she quickly cut me off, having clearly already decided that she was having none of it.

"And to think," she spat venomously, "it was only the other day that I was telling people how far you'd come since you joined the department. And now you go and pull a stunt like this."

And with that, our working relationship ended the way it began: with disappointment and antipathy. Saint George of England I most certainly was not; The Dragon Lady had set me alight, chewed me up, and spat me out. But at least, thank God, my time as her junior was finally over – and I could now rest safe in the knowledge I would never have to set eyes upon that withered, merciless face ever again.

Or could I...?

YOU HAVE THE COPYRIGHT
TO REMAIN SILENT

In between bouts fighting my very own sour-faced dragon, a depressingly large part of my O&G attachment was spent in the 'delightful' company of Mr Jonathan Parker, a snide, arrogant oddity of a man, whose peculiar character quirks ensured that none of his colleagues would be likely to forget him in a hurry.

I quickly came to see Mr Parker as the kind of person who had spent their entire life trying to be part of the 'in' crowd, desperately wanting to rub shoulders with the cool kids, but whose efforts were ultimately undermined by their grasping, awkward sense of humour. This made many of the things Mr Parker said and did quietly cringing to those watching – even, for example, something as seemingly innocuous as dictating clinic letters for his long-suffering secretary, Julie.

"I have therefore pencilled this lady in to one of my follow-up clinics in four weeks' time. Many thanks, yours sincerely, etc.," Mr Parker said into his Dictaphone in his distinctive nasally voice. As he sat back in his chair in the theatre recovery room, mulling over the final line of the dictation he had just completed, he muttered under his breath, "Hmm, four weeks – now what day would that be?" He turned to me (as I worked on what felt like my four hundred and fifty-eighth patient discharge summary that day) and asked, "Ahmed, what day is the twenty-seventh of this month?"

"It's a Monday, Mr Parker," I replied without hesitation. I just so happened to know that because the twenty-seventh of that particular month is my birthday (and that year it thankfully marked the first day of a very long overdue week off).

A smirk spread across Mr Parker's face. "Oh? And how did you happen to know that off the top of your head? Would that happen to be when you'll finally be having that first date with that *special someone*?" He chuckled to himself, marvelling at his own hilarity (there was, at that time, no special someone in my life) before returning to his dictations.

"Next patient: Pamela Lowton, date of birth 20/04/80. Dear GP, I have discussed this lady with my colleagues, and blah blah blah blah blah. Many thanks, yours sincerely, etc." Mr Parker paused before adding, "Julie, please remind me to actually discuss this lady with my colleagues."

Above all though, Mr Parker was the kind of person who positively revelled in the position of power and authority that his consultant role afforded him. In his mind, he was quite simply better than you, and he had absolutely no scruples when it came to rubbing it in your face. This is a man who, in theatre, would stand back from the operating table at the end of surgery before throwing his arms wide, turning to one of the theatre nurses and loudly demanding, "Disrobe me!" The nurse would dutifully obey while Mr Parker stood there smugly, looking like some kind of bizarre cross between a low-rent Jesus Christ (clearly taking the whole God complex thing far too literally), and Michael Jackson in the music video for

Earth Song.

I had, of course, come across consultants with a God complex before. The most notorious culprits in that particular hospital were actually the Cardiothoracic surgeons, though the Vascular team gave them a pretty good run for their money. Indeed, one particular Cardiothoracic consultant had such an overinflated opinion of himself that he would, quite literally, walk onto the wards and proclaim, "Fear not, everyone, God is here." However, even they never took the frankly baffling step Mr Parker did: copyrighting his own patient consent forms.

"Ahmed, go get me a JP10 form, would you?" Mr Parker asked me during my very first Gynae clinic with him. "Sharon will show you where to find one." I obediently made my way over to the main clinic office where Sharon, one of the ANPs, was working on the computer.

"Hi, Sharon," I said. "Mr Parker asked me to get him a JP10 form. Could you please show me where they are?"

"Of course," Sharon replied, before proceeding to rifle through one of the nearby drawers.

"Sharon, I'm sorry to ask, but – what *is* a JP10 form? I've not come across one before."

"Well," Sharon said, as she produced a piece of paper from the drawer and handed it to me, "it's just a patient consent form, really. Mr Parker gets all his patients to sign one in clinic before adding their name to the theatre waiting list." I thought I could sense a faint smirk creep across her face as she added, "All the other consultants just use standard consent forms, but Mr Parker insists on using his own."

I looked at the form Sharon had just passed to me. At the bottom, in small but bold writing, appeared the words: JP10

Form, Version 3 – © Jonathan Parker, 2010

To this day, I genuinely have no idea why Mr Parker had one day decided to amend the standard hospital consent form, slap his name on it, and then go to the frankly absurd effort of copyrighting it. Did he actually make any money from them? Was he so protective of his 'inspired' changes (not that there were many) to the standard form that he just couldn't bear the thought of anyone else freely adopting them? Or was it simply, as I suspect, the ultimate ego trip for a consultant who had such a high opinion of himself it would make Kanye West blush? By copyrighting his own consent forms, patients were essentially not just 'signing their life away' – they were specifically signing it over to *him*.

Within the O&G department, Mr Parker's capacity to be sarcastic, petty and/or demeaning when things displeased him was also well-known. I myself got off somewhat lightly in this regard (possibly due to my junior status), though wasn't fully immune. I remember going into his office once to ask for some advice on a patient of his, whose swab result had come back positive for a particular type of bacterial infection.

"Mr Parker," I began, "I just wanted to ask you about a patient of yours whom I saw earlier in antenatal clinic. Her vaginal swab result has come back positive for beta haemolytic streptococcus."

"Oh no!" Mr Parker replied sarcastically, as he put a closed fist in his mouth. "Whatever will we do?!" It was exactly the kind of dismissive, unhelpful retort everyone knew to expect from him if you asked a question he deemed to be irritating, or just plain unworthy of his copy-written time.

The registrars had it much worse. In theatre, Mr Parker

would often just sit and observe (at an uncomfortably close distance) as his registrar performed the operation. His 'feedback' would mainly take the form of anally critiquing the vast majority of whatever his junior colleague was doing. On one occasion, I even saw Mr Parker, mid-procedure, slap the hand of his very experienced registrar with a brusque, "No, not like that!" merely because she was holding some forceps a touch too low for his liking.

My number one abiding memory of Mr Parker, however, and perhaps the ultimate example of his petty childishness, was an incident that occurred during one of his Gynae clinics. I walked into the main clinic office (to retrieve the notes for my next patient) to see Mr Parker, mid-rant, addressing Sharon the ANP.

"And do you know perhaps the worst referral I've ever had, Sharon? It was a couple of months ago, in fact. A GP referred this morbidly obese woman to see me, and she stank. I mean, proper *stank*. She stank up my room, the corridor, the reception area; worse still, it took days before the smell finally went, presumably after a couple of deep cleans. Well, I decided to punish this GP for having referred this woman to me in the first place – and so, in my clinic letter, I sarcastically wrote: "Dear GP, my sincerest thanks for referring this forty-two-year-old malodorous woman to my clinic."

Suddenly noticing my presence, Mr Parker turned round and said, "Ahmed, you wanna be a GP, don't you? Well, I'll say this: if you do, then don't you dare ever refer a patient to me who stinks as much as that one did!"

Ah, Mr Parker, if only I still lived in that part of the country, you can all but guarantee I would have made a special point of referring all my so-called malodourous Gynae patients just to you – that *special someone*.

NEVER SAY ALAN AGAIN

One of the many saving graces of my four months spent under the wrinkled thumb of The Dragon Lady was the O&G registrars. They were, almost without exception, a friendly and supportive group of senior colleagues (though their near universal admiration of Ms O'Brien continues to baffle me no end). One of my favourite registrars was Mafu, a kind, gentle giant of a man, who was originally from Tonga. Calm under pressure and softly-spoken, he had the kind of voice you could happily listen to for hours. For some reason, however, though he and I always got on well, he became almost intractably convinced quite early on in the rotation that my name was, in fact, Alan.

As I mentioned earlier in this book, my parents are originally from the Middle East, and my own complexion is thus, unsurprisingly, fairly typically Arabic. Arabs, generally speaking, don't have names like Alan.

The first time I heard Mafu call me by that name, I assumed I had misheard him and so said nothing. The second time he said it, I actually did take a moment to correct his mistake, and politely explained that my name is in fact Ahmed. The very next time I saw Mafu, however, I was back to being Alan – and at that point, in characteristically British fashion, decided to just silently go along with the mistaken moniker. And so it was that the name stuck – and I mean like superglue.

At one stage, I honestly wondered if Mafu was, frankly, just quietly taking the piss. One day, about two months into the attachment, I helped assist Mafu with a routine caesarean section. Once it was over (mum and baby both thankfully well), I headed back to labour ward, only to be bleeped by Mafu just minutes later.

"Oh hello, Alan," Mafu said (in his unmistakeable, mellifluous Polynesian accent). "I'm just writing up the notes for that lady whose caesarean you assisted me with, and wanted to make sure I spelled your full name correctly in the operation notes."

This is it, I thought, *my chance to finally be rid of 'Alan' for ever*! I happily, and carefully, spelled out my name for Mafu in full, including my given name: A – H – M – E – D.

As the faint sound of hasty, scratchy biro-writing ceased in the background, Mafu cheerfully replied, "Okay – thanks, Alan," and hung up the phone.

Ironically, my last shift on labour ward was with Mafu. About an hour into the shift, we reviewed a patient together who had just been admitted to the Early Pregnancy Assessment Unit, after which Mafu asked me to carry out some routine blood tests for her.

"I'll get right on it," I replied.

"Okay – thanks, Ahmed."

As I turned away from Mafu, I suddenly stopped dead in my tracks. Had I heard him right? As I instinctively slowly turned back towards him, I could see that Mafu had an unmistakeably sheepish look on his face.

"I've been calling you the wrong name for the past four

months, haven't I?" he asked embarrassedly.

I genuinely couldn't think of anything to say, and so just quietly nodded, a sheepish look now plastered across my face too. We stood in silence for a moment, before parting ways. That was the last time I ever saw him.

As I walked away, I couldn't help but smile. Here we were, an Arab and a Tongan, and yet our mutual awkward shyness had been so quintessentially British it bordered on cliché.

Kind of like the name Alan, really.

STING IN THE DRAGON'S TAIL

And so it was over: my first year as a junior doctor had come to an end. In my case that meant not just another change of specialty, but also a change in hospital, and even a change in city as I entered my Foundation Year 2 (FY2) year. I soon discovered though, that the ghosts of my FY1 year had not yet been laid to rest...

Around a month after I'd finished my O&G rotation and moved on to pastures new, I was at the (sadly now defunct) three-day V music festival with some friends of mine. On the first day there, I received an unexpected phone call from Ranjit, who had (God help him) succeeded me as Ms O'Brien's FY1. Before I had left O&G, I had attempted to show Ranjit the ropes during his pre-rotation shadowing, just as an outgoing FY1 had done for me during my shadowing period in Cardiology a year earlier. I also gave him my mobile number and told him he could ring me should he have any queries, an offer he inadvertently chose to take me up on a few hours after my arrival at the festival.

I excused myself from my friends' company and took the call. His queries were straightforward enough, but towards the end of the conversation he must've picked up on the escalating noise in the background, and asked me where I was.

"Oh, I'm at V Festival," I replied cheerfully. "I'm here for the full three-day weekend with a couple of mates."

"Oh, how funny!" Ranjit replied. "I was in theatre with Ms O'Brien yesterday, and she told me that she'd be spending the weekend at V Festival too! Anyway, hope you have fun!"

Within an instant, Ranjit had unwittingly ruined my weekend. I never did actually run into Ms O'Brien at V Festival, but the heightened sense of paranoia Ranjit's words instilled in me for the duration of that entire three-day weekend meant the damage was already done.

God, I *hate* dragons.

PART IV

TRAUMA & ORTHOPAEDICS

A LITTLE MORE ORTHOPAEDICS, A LITTLE LESS TRAUMA, PLEASE

I think it's fair to say that between my four months in vascular surgery, and the four months of Obs & Gynae which immediately followed it, I was definitely starting to miss doing medical (as opposed to surgical) rotations by the time I began my FY2 year. I'll be the first to admit that surgery is not my personal forte, on top of which (as you'll have no doubt gleaned from reading Parts II and III of this book) my experience with surgeons during my FY1 year had, for the most part, not exactly been a stellar one. And so it was that, brimming with surgical ennui, I began the first rotation of my FY2 year: four months in Trauma & Orthopaedics (or T&O for short). As you can imagine, I was *thrilled*.

My ending up in that job was, to be fair, actually a somewhat calculated move on my part. I had become increasingly aware as I progressed through my FY1 year that General Practice was indeed the specialty for which I wanted to apply, something I would have to do just a few months into my FY2 year. Thus, as much as possible, my main aim for FY2 was to try to complete as balanced and varied a series of rotations as possible before the end of that year, and what I hoped would be the subsequent start of my time in GP training (subject to both a successful application and entrance exams).

Unlike many of my contemporaries working elsewhere in the country, myself and the other doctors in the geographical deanery where I did my FY1 training had only been allocated our three, first year rotations when we began working as junior doctors, as opposed to all six of the rotations we would end up doing over the course of our first two foundation years. Consequently, partway through our FY1 year, we had to submit a fresh batch of applications for FY2. However, though you had to remain within the same deanery, you could choose to relocate to another hospital within that area if you so wished – and so it was with me. Before I knew it, within the space of a single day one August, I had packed my life into my trusty Honda Civic, and relocated from a large city to a tiny town a forty-five minute drive away, in the process downsizing from working at a big teaching hospital to a much smaller so-called district general hospital (DGH).

What had attracted me to the move was not so much the change in hospital (though that did afford me the enviable training opportunity to practise medicine in a different kind of working environment), but the placements that this DGH had to offer. Specifically, I was intrigued by one set of rotations in particular: T&O, General Practice, and community Psychiatry (in that order). For a budding GP, such a combination seemed like an invaluable learning opportunity, one that would surely put me in good stead for the formal GP training that was hopefully to come. What it would mean, however, was going straight into yet another surgical rotation – my third in succession. I was very much aware that, by the time the

T&O attachment was over, I would be starting my very first GP placement having not done medicine for over a year. But I reasoned it was a price worth paying if it meant I could do those three rotations as an FY2.

And so it was that, with my FY1 year now behind me, I began my temporary career as an orthopod.

DIAL 'O' FOR 'OBSEQUIOUS'

Compared to my two previous surgical jobs, T&O did have one major advantage, which became apparent almost immediately: I actually quite *liked* my boss. Especially after four months spent in the less than delightful company of the dreaded Dragon Lady, this was nothing short of a minor miracle.

My consultant, John Franks (who also happened to be head of the Orthopaedic department) was, on the surface, a very unassuming man in his early fifties. Admittedly, like many Orthopaedic consultants, he occasionally liked to put on a bit of a laddish façade, especially in the operating room when chatting with the theatre staff. On one occasion, he even joked with one of the Anaesthetists about having attended wild socials that had been likened to 'bunga bunga' parties, a term coined by former (hedonistic) Italian prime minister Silvio Berlusconi to describe the debauched soirées he would throw at his private villa. But, unlike with many other surgeons of his ilk, you always intrinsically knew that such stories were all front and no substance.

At his core, he was a kind and supportive boss, who seemed genuinely keen on ensuring me and the other junior doctors got the most educationally out of our attachment. He was also someone who you knew had your back. I shall always remember an incident in which another of the consultants, Mr Pike, was unashamedly reprimanding me on the ward, prompting Mr Franks to chime in and defend me, something for which I was immeasurably grateful. But more on that later...

He was also a very intelligent, methodical individual who very much knew his stuff – unless, of course, you handed him a heart tracing (ECG), in which case he would react in the exact same manner as all the other seniors in that department: with a look of abject horror. Passing him an ECG for one of his patients during the afternoon ward round one day, he even replied, "Urgh, get that away from me!" as though what I'd handed him was radioactive. Yes, I soon learned that this was just another one of those surgical clichés which really do hold true.

In spite of his affable nature, you would always sense a slight sadness behind Mr Franks's eyes; indeed, he often looked like a man who you suspected held the weight of the world on his shoulders. Part of this, it transpired, was a sense of frustration towards the hospital itself. At the end of the day, this was not, I sensed, where he truly wanted to be. DGHs such as his were often restricted when it came to money and personnel, and I always thought Mr Franks secretly would have much rather been working at a large, inner city teaching hospital. To be fair to him, when the hospital you work at frequently boasts that its MS-DOS-based computer system is 'revolutionary', but then neglects to mention this was only true when it was installed in 1996 (and that it hasn't been significantly updated in more than fifteen years), it isn't exactly a great sign.

"Do you know, Ahmed," Mr Franks solemnly told me one day, "when I started at this hospital, it was ranked as the worst in the country. I've worked here for almost twenty years now, and all the hospital can really say it's achieved in that time is that it's now only ranked as the *third* worst."

I strongly suspected it was this inherent sense of dissatisfaction with his job role which explained why, aside from the odd moment of false bravado, I never really ever saw Mr Franks get fired up or truly energised by anything; anything, of course, apart from his visits to the infamous Rose Suite.

The Orthopaedic department was spread out across three wards: C1, C2 and the Rose Suite. Now, if the third item in that list sounds conspicuously different to the other two, it's because it was. All the NHS patients were almost exclusively housed on wards C1 and C2, while all the private patients went upstairs to the Rose Suite.

It's fair to say that, much like the Vascular surgeons I had worked alongside for four months as an FY1, the orthopods in our department did not exactly have a reputation for being the most compassionate individuals when it came to their bedside manner with patients. I soon discovered, however, that this only really held true for the NHS patients; when it came to the private patients, it was an entirely different social ballgame. To watch one of the Orthopaedic consultants during their ward rounds on C1 and 2 was typically an exercise in observed lofty, impatient boredom. However, as soon as the consultants headed up to the Rose Suite, it was as though an invisible switch had abruptly been flicked in their brains, and their demeanour underwent a complete one hundred and eighty. All of a sudden, they were jovial, thorough, and attentive, sometimes to the point of being downright fawning. And Mr Franks – a man for whom I otherwise held a great deal of respect – was sadly no exception.

When it came to their private patients, suddenly no job was too lowly or menial for the consultants to do themselves. Unlike their NHS patients, they were always conspicuously (and unusually) particular about what they would allow their juniors to do for the private patients under their care on the Rose Suite. I soon figured out that the reason for this was because the consultants were being paid top dollar by these patients to look after them, and thus it was very important to the consultants that they not only went the extra mile for their private patients, but that they be *seen* to be doing so as well. I guess that is the kind of reputation that only money can buy.

I remember once being asked – with unusual trepidation, and in an almost subservient manner – by one of the consultants to assist him in theatre with the hip replacement for one of his private patients, as the registrar who was supposed to have been helping him had gone off sick that day. During the operation itself, I was very much aware that my every move was being watched and scrutinised, and I was given more guidance and direction when it came to performing my (fairly basic) assistant tasks than I had ever been before or since. After the operation, the consultant thanked me for assisting him, and even shook my hand – the one and only time this ever happened in the entirety of my time on any surgical rotation.

As I mentioned, Mr Franks was not immune to this type of behaviour. One of the simplest but commonest jobs the juniors would be asked to do when on call would be to prescribe an appropriate dose of the blood thinning drug Warfarin for those patients who were taking it (the prescribed dose would typically vary fairly regularly based on the patient's most recent blood test results). I shall never forget my surprise during one particular Sunday on call when I was bleeped by the Rose Suite to come up later that afternoon and prescribe that evening's Warfarin dose for a particular patient, only for the ward to call back later to say that this would no longer be necessary. When I asked why, they explained that Mr Franks had prescribed the Warfarin for the gentleman in question, who was his patient. For a consultant to trouble him or herself with such a straightforward, relatively banal task would have been strange in itself – but I subsequently learned that Mr Franks had actually driven to the hospital from home, on a Sunday, on his day off, purely to prescribe the Warfarin. And had then promptly driven home again.

When I would ponder the way in which the consultants treated their private patients, my mind kept coming back to the same, inescapable thought: if the NHS patients just one floor below only knew how much more attentive the care their Rose Suite contemporaries were receiving really was, they would've been up in arms. And who could've blamed them? I'm not naïve enough to fail to realise that paying to go private will always open certain doors that would otherwise remain closed to you within the confines of a free, state-run healthcare service – but it was the gross inequity of the consultants' attitude that really got to me. After all, if it was your loved one lying in a hospital bed, you would surely want their consultant to be just as invested in their care as in the care of any of their other patients, regardless of whether they were on the first, second or tenth floor of the hospital. But I guess, even for someone as otherwise decent as Mr Franks, the old adage invariably holds true: money talks.

NIGHT FEVER

Night shifts on T&O were a decidedly mixed bag. Though some shifts were actually relatively straightforward, these were unfortunately very much in the minority. This was not surprising given that, between the hours of 9:00 p.m. and 8:00 a.m. the following morning, the responsibilities of the junior doctor on call for T&O included (but were not limited to):

• Looking after all fifty-odd Orthopaedic patients (by which I mean *approximately* fifty and not that they were all strange people), spread across at least the aforementioned three wards (not including any so-called outlying wards where Orthopaedic patients would occasionally be located), and doing everything from menial prescription tasks to urgent reviews of those patients who were critically ill;

• Clerking in the new Orthopaedic arrivals in A&E. Everyone, from people involved in serious road traffic collisions to (and this is true) a twenty-one-year-old partygoer with a broken finger, who rocked up to hospital at 4:00 a.m. after having dislocated his ring finger while ill-advisedly trying to karate chop a swan-shaped ice sculpture in order to impress his girlfriend (she was, I can assure you from the murderous look on her face as she sat next to him in the A&E cubicle, most definitely *not* impressed);

• Assisting the Orthopaedic registrar in theatre during emergency surgeries;

• Ensuring the following day's emergency theatre list/running order was up to date, and that everyone on it had had the necessary consent paperwork/bloods done;

• Filing (and, if necessary, actioning) any unseen/unfiled blood test and imaging results (which had been done for both inpatients and, frustratingly, even outpatients as well);

• Writing up the discharge paperwork for patients for whom this had not been completed by the day team.

Now, it's the last of these responsibilities that really used to irk me.

As you can imagine from the above list, there was a *lot* you were expected to do whilst on call overnight, on top of which, you were predominantly left to your own devices during your eleven-plus hour shift. Yes, there was an on call Orthopaedic registrar at night as well but, barring any emergencies that came in in the dead of night, they mostly tended to go home shortly after 10:00 p.m., accessible only by phone until their return shortly before 8:00 a.m. the next morning. I can't say I blamed them one bit; after all, the registrars typically also did a full day's shift on the days immediately before and after their night shift, and so if you called and woke them up in the middle of the night, it better be for a damn good reason. The end result, however, was that the night shifts could end up being pretty relentless for the junior doctor, and it might only take one critically ill patient on the ward or one especially complex A&E admission to pretty much make your night shift a bit of a write-off.

In the midst of all the above responsibilities, the very last thing on your mind at 3:00 a.m. was completing the discharge summary for a patient who had actually already left the hospital several hours earlier. Most people, you'd think, would understand that.

But Mr Lomas was not most people.

I can honestly say I have never met anyone quite like Mr Lomas. He was a man who screamed contradictions at every turn; he had a broad smile, but a lecherous laugh that would even make Sid James (of *Carry On* fame) squirm; he had an arrogance in stark contrast to his alleged poor surgical reputation (which was, if the rumour mill was to be believed, the reason he had ended up at this particular small DGH in the first place); and though he was incredibly tall in stature, the amount of respect and compassion he displayed towards colleagues was often miniscule. On this last point, it was undoubtedly the way he treated his registrar, Mr Pelios, I found especially distasteful.

Mr Pelios was an incredibly kind, intelligent and gentle man, who was always generous with his time if you needed any help and support. Unlike many others within that T&O department, he also, refreshingly, entirely lacked a chip on his shoulder, despite the fact he had actually been a consultant Orthopaedic surgeon within the army in his native Greece (with complicated issues relating to the recognition of certain international exam qualifications being the sole reason he did

121

not hold an equivalent surgical grade immediately after moving to the UK). As to why, then, Mr Pelios was so frequently a target of Mr Lomas's open critiques, I will never know – though unabashed jealousy has always been my prevailing theory.

Mr Lomas would always turn up to work sometime between 6:00 and 6:30 a.m. - i.e. at least ninety minutes early (none of the other consultants, it should be said, ever did this). Mr Pelios would turn up to work just after 7:00 a.m. which, again, none of the other registrars ever did. However, simply due to the fact he would rock up to work forty-five minutes or so *after* his boss, he was consistently branded lazy and workshy by Mr Lomas. Indeed, despite Mr Pelios being both well-liked and widely respected within the department, I never once heard Mr Lomas extend him a compliment. In fact, Mr Lomas's theatre lists would frequently descend into tirades of entirely undeserved verbal abuse against his registrar. To my shock (and in a way that would bring back uncomfortable memories of Mr Parker from my O&G rotation), you would even sometimes see Mr Lomas physically hit Mr Pelios on the arm, mid-operation, if the latter had done something to displease his boss. My only explanation for Mr Pelios's remarkably high levels of tolerance for his largely intolerable boss is that he had, presumably, been forced to deal with a lot worse in the Greek army.

As I alluded to above, Mr Lomas was very much a creature of habit. At 6:30 a.m. on the dot, the junior doctor who'd been on call overnight was expected to meet him in his office, help him update that day's emergency theatre list (the so-called 'trauma list'), and then accompany him on a brief ward round. Now, this was not a ward round for the patients who'd been admitted overnight (which surely would have made infinitely more sense); no, this was a ward round of Mr Lomas's *own* patients, the vast majority of whom said junior doctor would likely have had zero involvement with during their night shift. Why Mr Lomas couldn't simply wait until after the 8:00 a.m. morning team meeting to do this, accompanied by his own junior doctor (who actually did know the patients, and would be responsible for doing any of the big jobs arising from the ward round), was never entirely clear to me. I came to the conclusion that – like many of the Vascular surgeons I'd worked with – Mr Lomas simply saw reviewing his patients as a chore he wanted to dispense with as early as physically possible each morning.

Now, I'm used to surgical ward rounds being brisk, but Mr Lomas's rounds happened at such breakneck speed they bordered on the absurd. For starters, you already came into them very much on the back foot since, in addition to already being exhausted from the stress of the night shift, you didn't know most (if any) of his patients, nor which beds or even wards they were in. Add to this the fact that Mr Lomas would often spend less than thirty seconds with each (typically still half-asleep) patient, and you'd get a ward round so confused and frenetic that it frequently resembled a Benny Hill chase sequence. Half the time, you wouldn't even have had the chance to locate and retrieve the patient's notes before Mr Lomas had summarily moved onto the next one (he would never wait for you). This once gave rise to an entry (penned by my junior doctor colleague, Adam) in a set of patient notes that still ranks amongst my all-time favourites:

Ward Round Mr Lomas, 18th October, 6:45 a.m.

?

Dr Adam Collins, FY2

I think the question mark says it all, really.

When you were 'summoned' (bleeped) to meet Mr Lomas in his office at 6:30 a.m. each morning, he would always ask you the same two questions before you even sat down to begin helping him update the trauma list:

1) "Have you filed all the results?" and,

2) "Have you completed all the discharge summaries?"

I was told when I started the job that, no matter how busy or stressful a night shift you'd just had, your answer to the above two questions had better always be yes.

Sadly, however, this just simply wasn't always possible. It didn't matter so much on a weekend (i.e. when Mr Lomas wasn't in, save for the rare instances when he himself was on call), as the other consultants never asked you about results or discharge letters, and probably didn't much care. But on a weekday? Your answer to those two questions *always* mattered, because Mr Lomas never forgot to ask.

I remember one particular Tuesday night on call shift (my second in a run of four nights) that had been especially busy, due to a combination of multiple overnight Orthopaedic admissions via A&E, and a few very sick patients on the wards. There were also, unfortunately, *eleven* outstanding discharge summaries that needed to be done. I had, somehow, managed to find time at around 5:00 a.m. to complete four of them before being urgently called away. But in a hectic shift that had barely even afforded me the opportunity for a toilet break, I simply hadn't had the time to start on the remaining seven by 6:30 a.m. And frankly, they simply hadn't been a priority for me anyway, a rationalisation I stand by even now. I mean come on, it's not like the GPs had been up all night waiting for said discharge letters to come through.

I reasoned in my head that if I simply explained to Mr Lomas how busy the night shift had been (but how, in spite of that, I had still at least managed to complete four of the letters), he might be sympathetic and just let the matter slide. After all, the discharge summaries were surely not the highest priority job, and the day team (who should've really done the letters anyway) would be arriving in just ninety short minutes. *It'll be fine*, I thought.

I thought wrong.

"So, Ahmed – have you filed all the results?"

"Yes, Mr Lomas," I replied like an obedient schoolboy.

"And have you completed all the discharge summaries?"

I paused.

"I'm afraid not, Mr Lomas," I said awkwardly.

He scowled; I perspired. I calmly tried to explain why I hadn't had the time to finish them all. He simply didn't care. In hindsight, knowing him, I probably should have seen it coming.

"After the morning meeting, Ahmed, you're going to stay behind until you've completed every one of those discharge summaries – and I'm going to check to make sure that you do."

And so it was that I didn't leave the hospital that morning until just past 10:30 a.m., over two hours after my shift was supposed to have finished. I can only hope that my fellow junior doctors didn't catch sight of me silently cursing them with my eyes that morning as I diligently sat at a computer and finished all seven outstanding letters, my brain sluggish and dulled through stress, fatigue and frustration.

As I finally departed the ward that morning, exhausted and dejected (and dreading the thought of having to do it all again in just over ten hours), I passed Mr Lomas's closed office door and glared at it in silence for a moment. In that instant, my discombobulated thoughts aligned perfectly with those of my colleague Adam during his infamous early morning frenetic ward round with Mr Lomas. Quite simply, I just thought: ?

DON'T TELL HIM, PIKE!

Forgive me, once again, for the impending use of colourful language, but there really is no other way to say it. Within the T&O department, with all its peculiar individuals of questionable character, Mr Pike had a well-earned reputation as a bit of a mean-spirited bastard – and that's me putting it mildly (my colleague Adam once even referred to Mr Pike as a 'C u next Tuesday'. Ahem). This was a fact I discovered for myself (in no uncertain terms) around two months into the job.

In many ways, I'd been fortunate. During my time in T&O up to that point my interactions with Mr Pike had been minimal. In addition, his FY2 junior was a quiet woman who wasn't prone to bouts of idle gossip about her boss. As a result, I knew surprisingly little about this man, even halfway through my attachment. All of that was to change one fateful Saturday morning.

In the way that life sometimes is, circumstances had lulled me into a false sense of security that morning. After all, this being a Saturday – and my having just done the night shift – meant one glorious, wondrous thing: this was one of those enviable, once-in-a-blue-moon night shifts that we all coveted: one in which you didn't have to trundle off to Mr Lomas's office at 6:30 a.m. for his heart-sinking early morning meeting.

I felt like I was on vacation.

The night itself had been fairly reasonable; not too many new A&E admissions, and only a mercifully small number of patients on the wards who had become acutely unwell overnight. I was up to date with my on call jobs, feeling good, and looking forward to a well-deserved day's slumber.

Your final on call responsibility when you were on nights was to attend the 8:00 a.m. morning team meeting, to go through the upcoming trauma list with that day's on call consultant, and then accompany said consultant on the so-called 'post-take' ward round, when you would review the new patients who had been admitted overnight.

I had gone through and updated the trauma list prior to the 8:00 a.m. meeting (as I normally did), ensuring that I was up to speed on the clinical details and, crucially, indications for surgery for the patients on it. The one exception was a lady called Patricia Atlas, a seventy-three-year-old elective patient who had been added to the trauma list the day before by Mr Aziz, one of the other consultants. I had assumed (not unreasonably, I felt) that – having added Mrs Atlas to the list himself – Mr Aziz had already discussed the case in advance with Mr Pike. Sadly, just like with Mr Lomas and the discharge summaries, I had once again assumed wrongly.

Cut to the morning meeting. Having systematically gone through all the other patients on the trauma list, we came, inevitably, to the last person in the running order: Mrs Atlas.

"And who's this last lady on the list?" Mr Pike enquired, "Mrs Atlas?"

"She," I replied, "is Mrs Patricia Atlas, a seventy-three-year-old lady on ward C1. She's the elective patient who has come in today at the request of Mr Aziz."

There followed an uncomfortable silence. From the expectant look on his face, it was clear Mr Pike was after more details – and, eventually, I made a fumbling attempt to fill the void I had unwittingly created.

"Did... did Mr Aziz not discuss the case with you, Mr Pike?"

"No, no he did not," Mr Pike replied matter-of-factly. "So, why don't you tell me all about her?"

There was another awkward silence. Suddenly, I became very aware that all the eyes in the room (including Mr Pike's, his registrar's, and those of the theatre staff) were focused squarely on me. There was sadly nowhere to hide.

"I'm afraid I don't know Mrs Atlas's clinical history," I replied in a small and rather sheepish voice. "I had assumed that Mr Aziz had added her name to the trauma list after discussing it with you, Mr Pike."

What followed yet another uncomfortable silence was a five minute, entirely unapologetic rant by Mr Pike that was nothing short of devastating. In a restrained yet stern tone of voice (the lack of any shouting somehow made everything he said ten times worse), he proceeded to tell me in no uncertain terms, in front of a room full of people, how thoroughly unprofessional, and simply unforgivable, my lack of knowledge on Mrs Atlas truly was. His diatribe against me eventually morphed into a tirade about junior doctors in general, one which left you with the distinct impression he'd just been itching for an opportunity to air these clearly long-held views.

"That's the problem with so many junior doctors like you," Mr Pike opined. "No work ethic, no sense of professionalism, and a complete unwillingness to actually prove yourself to be a conscientious team player. Frankly, if this is the kind of attitude you bring to work, then I don't know why we even bother having the junior doctors at these morning meetings. It's a complete waste of everybody's time. To be honest, we might as well just have the nurses in here instead. They may not be able to actually tell you much beyond, 'Oh, patient had a poo this morning', but at least they're doing their job properly. It's simply *unacceptable*. I mean, don't you agree?" He turned to the others in the meeting room. Not one of them had the faintest idea what to say.

What followed was possibly the most excruciating post-take ward round of my entire medical career. On every ward, in every patient bay, and in front of practically every passing member of staff (and even a few patients), Mr Pike took absolutely every opportunity to criticise, belittle and demean both me, and junior doctors in general.

Up on the Rose Suite, we happened to run into my consultant, Mr Franks, who (in an entirely unsurprising display) had come in on the weekend, on his day off, to review one of his private patients. Spotting yet another opportunity to dig in the proverbial boot, Mr Pike proceeded to loudly complain to his colleague about what a terrible morning he'd been having, due to the "incompetence of these junior doctors."

Glancing from Mr Pike to myself and back to Mr Pike again, Mr Franks attempted to lightly dismiss his colleague's criticisms.

"Oh come on, Bob," Mr Franks said jovially. "Now, I've worked with young Ahmed here for the better part of two months, and I actually think he's a really good foundation year doctor."

Seeing my boss stick up for me was an unexpected moment that truly meant a lot to me – but sadly, Mr Pike remained unmoved.

"Well, you could've fooled me, John," Mr Pike shot back, "because I've been on a ward round with him for the past hour, and I've yet to see a single shred of anything remotely good."

So, what's the lesson here? Should I have taken the time to read through Mrs Atlas's notes prior to that 8:00 a.m. meeting, just in case Mr Aziz had (as turned out to be the case) failed to tell Mr Pike why, exactly, he had put her on his colleague's Saturday trauma list? With the benefit of hindsight, absolutely, yes. But was Mr Pike's response unnecessarily harsh, not to mention arguably unprofessional (especially the unashamedly public way in which he chose to air his grievances)? Undoubtedly so.

Someone a bit more thick-skinned than I would perhaps have been able to simply shrug off what Mr Pike had said, chalk it up to experience, and promptly move on with their life. But I am someone who, for better or worse, takes things very much to heart, and Mr Pike's repeated assertions that I was unconscientious, unprofessional and generally incompetent genuinely cut deep (to the point that this incident still lingers vividly in my memory, years later). It was also yet more proof, if any were needed, that I was simply not cut out to be a surgeon – or, at the very least, that I just wasn't cut out to be a mean-spirited bastard. Either way, I silently thanked God as I finally left work that morning, exhausted, broken and humiliated, that my days working in hospital were mercifully numbered.

PART V

RESPIRATORY, GERIATRICS, AND PAEDIATRICS

LEVELLING UP

Once my time in T&O had (jubilantly) come to an end, there was a distinct shift in the tone of my FY2 year. For the first time, I began doing attachments that were based either exclusively or predominantly in the community, and this was both a marked and welcome change of pace after sixteen straight months spent working in hospital medicine. The latter two thirds of my time in FY2 consisted of a four-month stint in General Practice, followed by four months in community Psychiatry. Though I knew my time working on hospital wards had not yet come to an end, those eight months were certainly a much needed respite of (near) normality after the rigours of everything that had come before.

Typically partway through your FY2 year you apply for what is termed specialty training. As opposed to the more mixed rotations you do as an FY1 and FY2, your specialty training (as the name suggests) is specifically geared towards the particular area of medicine or surgery in which you intend to end up specialising – everything from Anaesthetics to Urology, by way of General Practice, Pathology, Psychiatry and everything else in between. The duration of specialty training varies depending on the specialty itself, but is typically around six or seven years (excluding any 'life' factors that prolong it, like part-time working, maternity leave, etc.). General Practice, interestingly, is actually the shortest specialty training scheme of all, spanning just three years (at the time of writing, at least). So, in theory, you could go from qualifying as a doctor to working as a fully-fledged GP in only five short years, and indeed, this is what ultimately happened with me. Of those three years of GP training, approximately half is spent working in hospital medicine, with the other half spent in General Practice itself.

But before all that, of course, you have to physically be accepted onto the specialty scheme in which you wish to train. Fortunately, my application was successful. I did well in the entrance exams, and just a few short months later I was on the move again, this time relocating to another DGH, and back to the mean old streets of East Anglia where I had grown up.

The three years of specialty training in General Practice are referred to as ST1, 2 and 3. The first two years – much like the foundation years – each consisted of three, four-month rotations: two in hospital medicine and one in General Practice. The third and final year, however, was based exclusively at a GP surgery. For me, my last four jobs in hospital medicine were to be Respiratory, Geriatrics (aka care of the elderly), A&E, and finally Paediatrics.

As I began my ST1 year, and reacclimatised myself to life working on the wards, I quickly discovered I was destined to come across at least a few more colourful characters before the final curtain would come down on my time in hospital medicine.

ST1 (RESPIRATORY): MISTAKEN IDENTITY (AKA ACTING RASHLY)

It is a truth universally acknowledged, that a man in possession of medical knowledge, must be in want of an acronym.

Given the sheer volume of facts and information we need to remember, I guess it's hardly surprising that medics love acronyms. Some of my favourites include INBOW (If No Better Or Worse), GET SMASHED (denoting the common causes of pancreatitis), and FOOSH (Fall Onto Out Stretched Hand), a typical mechanism of injury causing wrist fractures (and sadly not – as I once briefly hypothesised upon first seeing the acronym in a set of notes – a hilarious, *boing*-like sound effect describing the slapstick way in which said person slipped and fell). Another commonly used one is DANISH, which is designed to help doctors remember some of the signs that may indicate disease of the cerebellum (the part of the brain responsible for co-ordinating voluntary movements). The S in DANISH stands for slurred or staccato speech. Now, I was already familiar with the term staccato from my days learning the piano many moons ago (it essentially means to perform each note sharply and separately from the others), but had long been confused as to what exactly staccato *speech* sounded like. All of that changed the day I met my new boss in Respiratory medicine, Dr Shonde, a woman whose inimitable speech patterns must surely have led to the phrase 'staccato speech' being coined in the first place.

A fiercely intelligent, confident Afro-Caribbean woman in her forties, Dr Shonde spoke in such a way that each individual syllable was expressed in short, sharp utterances that made each sentence sound oddly disjointed. At first, I thought this was just how she spoke at work – some curious affectation designed to give her words more impact. However, I eventually discovered this was not the case at all.

At the end of each rotation, Dr Shonde used to invite all the junior doctors who had worked for her over the preceding few months to her house, and would cook them an end-of-attachment meal as a way of saying thank you for all their hard work.

"So what are you cooking, Dr Shonde?" I asked her as I stepped into her kitchen to grab myself a drink.

"*Well*, *Ah*med," she replied, "I *ho*pe you like *fish* – I'm making *sal*mon with *tartare* sauce."

This was just one of the humorous discoveries I made that evening. The other was that her dog, bless him, had Chronic Obstructive Pulmonary Disease (COPD). As a result, every time he walked into a room, he made a raspy breathing noise which, I'll be honest, made him sound like a gremlin. I shouldn't laugh really, but the fact that a Respiratory consultant owned a dog with a lung condition was inherently amusing to me. It couldn't help but make me wonder what other pets she had. A parrot with asthma? A cat with cystic fibrosis?

Dr Shonde could certainly take her work seriously, but more so she was very no-nonsense when it came to her responsibilities as an educator (she was in charge of helping all the core medical trainees prepare for their clinical exams). On alternate Thursday mornings, beginning at 7:45 a.m., she would put on a mandatory teaching session for all the junior doctors working in medical specialties, one you quickly learned *never* to be late for. Why? Because she kept a register of attendance for these morning sessions – and as soon as the session had begun, she would immediately replace the register with an alternate one specifically for latecomers. Appear on the late register more than once, and Dr Shonde would report you to your educational supervisor. Yes, when it came to teaching, this lady took no prisoners.

However, Dr Shonde also undoubtedly had a bit of a silly side to her. The very first morning we did a ward round with her, she assembled all the junior doctors together like expectant school children, and made the following announcement (in order to spare you all from any further irregular italicisation, you'll just have to imagine the following words spoken in her unique style of stop-start diction):

"Okay, team – this is what we're going to do. I want to make sure that we start each and every morning on a bright and positive note. So when we gather for ward rounds, I don't want to see any dour faces! I'm going to say, 'Good morning, team!' and you're going to reply, nice and cheerily, 'Good morning, Dr Shonde!' So – let's all give it a go, shall we? Good morning, team!"

"Good morning, Dr Shonde," came our somewhat muted, half-hearted reply.

Perhaps given our less than enthusiastic response, Dr Shonde's proposed junior school-esque morning exchange, rather unsurprisingly, failed to ever make an encore.

Dr Shonde's penchant for school-era antics didn't stop there. She was good friends with Dr Gregory, a Radiologist who would often attend the lung MDT meetings. When one of her fellow Respiratory consultants would read out the NHS number for the patient they wished to discuss (so that Dr Gregory could pull up said patient's images on the computer), Dr Shonde would often simultaneously whisper an entirely different set of digits in her friend's ear, much to Dr Gregory's chagrin, and to the amusement of the rest of us. It was in moments such as these that Dr Shonde would have an unmistakeable twinkle in her eye that no one could fail to notice.

My favourite story about Dr Shonde concerns a case of mistaken identity. During our end-of-rotation sign-off meeting, she recounted the story of Mr Jeffries, one of her elderly male patients, who had been under her care during his hospital admission with severe pneumonia some months earlier. Six weeks later, he had attended a follow-up appointment in Dr Shonde's outpatient clinic, flanked by his wife.

"Go on," Mrs Jeffries had insisted to her husband as the pair of them sat down, "tell Dr Shonde what you've been telling me over and over."

"Tell me what, sorry?" Dr Shonde had asked blankly.

With a loud sigh, Mrs Jeffries had continued. "Honestly, Dr Shonde, he's been banging on about this for the past six weeks. Go on, Stan – tell her."

"Well, Dr Shonde, it's like this," Mr Jeffries began. "As you know, when I was admitted here last month I was in a very bad way. I don't remember much of that first twenty-four hours, but I do know that I was on my way out. I do have one very clear memory from that first day, though – and it involves you, Dr Shonde."

Dr Shonde's curiosity very much piqued, Mr Jeffries had continued:

"So there I was, at death's door, and it's no exaggeration to say that I even started to see the light – when, all of a sudden, I was brought back to earth by a real-world angel. And in that moment, there – standing above me with a smile on her face – was Halle Berry herself!"

Sadly, any ego boost this story gave Dr Shonde was very much undone by another incident that occurred some months later – one which may have enjoyed a similar beginning but most certainly had a different outcome.

At the end of one particular Tuesday afternoon outpatient clinic appointment, a female patient in her seventies rose from her chair, put on her coat, and thanked Dr Shonde for her time. As she headed for the door, the patient turned back to Dr Shonde and, with a wry smile on her face, stated, "You know, Dr Shonde, I'm sure you get this all the time, but you really are the spitting image of someone very famous."

"Oh?" Dr Shonde replied cheerily. "And who's that?"

"Shirley Bassey."

For the record, Shirley Bassey is almost thirty years older than Halle Berry. I think it's fair to say that in that moment, having just had her likeness compared to someone almost four decades her senior, the trademark twinkle in Dr Shonde's eye was abruptly extinguished. I can imagine more than a few short, sharp utterances Dr Shonde would have loved nothing more than to express to that patient, but fortunately she thought better of it and sent the lady on her way. I do wonder though, if – with the door firmly closed – Dr Shonde may have silently given her patient the (cold) finger.

Now, if you thought that pun was bad, just wait till you hear what's coming in this next section...

Being an ST1 put me in the novel and curious position of no longer being the most junior person in my particular team (even as an FY2, none of the rotations I did involved working directly alongside an FY1 doctor on a regular basis). Our Respiratory team, however, included two FY1s – and they could not have been more different as people.

One of the FY1s, Tunde, a young man originally from the Congo, was polite, always respectful, and highly dedicated. If he needed to stay on the wards for an hour or two (or three) past his contracted hours in order to get all his jobs done (an all too common experience as a junior doctor working in hospital medicine) he would, without question. He would also frequently, almost instinctively, revert to calling me Dr Handy, despite my repeated insistences that he just call me Ahmed. I was, after all, only two years more senior than Tunde, and always saw the FY1s and FY2s as contemporaries rather than my juniors. Tunde once explained to me that in his native Congo, the hierarchy that exists within the world of hospital medicine is much more demonstrably apparent than it is in the UK, so to him, calling me Dr Handy was just a natural, ingrained way of showing respect to a doctor more senior than he.

The other FY1, Rana, was such a marked contrast to Tunde that I sometimes struggled to believe the two were actually contemporaries. Fearless, gobby, and undeniably frustrating at times, Rana carried herself with a confident swagger that belied her inexperience as a doctor, and with a near permanent pout that practically screamed, "I don't have time for this shit." If she resented having to stay late to finish her jobs, she'd tell you so in no uncertain terms, often in stark contrast to the naïve earnestness that many FY1s share. On one occasion, I saw her refuse to accept a patient from a consultant (in a different specialty) simply because she didn't agree with the clinical rationale for the transfer of care. Now, that'd be a gutsy thing for even a senior registrar to do, but it's no exaggeration to say that for an FY1 to do so was all but unheard of. Perhaps it's just me, but I would've never *dared* do such a thing as a junior doctor; rightly or wrongly, I would've considered such an act akin to professional suicide.

And yet, despite her devil-may-care attitude, in her quieter moments there was an undeniable vulnerability evident behind Rana's often brash exterior, which couldn't help but endear her to me. Though we didn't always see eye to eye (mainly when it came to our respective, somewhat conflicting, work ethics), she and I still got along pretty well, and eventually became good friends. As with all good friends, we'd sometimes affectionately poke fun at one another – and when it came to Rana, there was no easier target for that humour than the hopeless crush she had on one of the core medical trainees, Charlie.

Charlie was a handsome, confidant man in his late twenties, who had originally graduated from Cambridge University. He also had a long-term girlfriend which, unfortunately for Rana, essentially rendered him off limits. This, however, didn't stop Rana from practically swooning over Charlie every chance she got, often in the most unsubtle manner possible. Yes, it's fair to say that her unashamed crush on this good-looking posh boy wasn't exactly a state secret.

On one particular Friday, Rana and I both happened to be on call for the medical department. We started the day, like any other on call, by attending the morning handover meeting, during which the team who'd been on call overnight would let the incoming day team know about the patients who'd been admitted to hospital during the preceding twelve hours. The night shift junior doctor, who informally led the handover, was also expected to let the day shift consultant know about any patients who'd come in overnight, and been discharged home. On that day, the junior doctor leading handover just happened to be Charlie. Cue the typical sight of Rana hanging on his every word as he spoke.

One of the patients Charlie mentioned in his handover was a four-year-old girl whose parents had brought her into hospital after she'd eaten a strawberry for the first time, and then come out in a rash (though otherwise remained entirely well in herself). The medics had given the patient some Piriton, her skin improved, and she was then sent home. As the consultant bemoaned the inappropriateness of the girl's parents deciding to take their daughter to hospital for such a simple complaint, an unmistakeable smirk appeared on Charlie's face as he replied, "Yes, I suppose you could say that theirs was a rather *rash* decision."

Everybody in the room audibly groaned – everybody, that

is, except Rana, who giggled like a love-struck schoolgirl (and just a little *too* loudly) at Charlie's appalling pun. Quickly, all eyes in the room turned towards Rana, and she was soon confronted with a sea of bemused faces.

A few weeks later, word spread that Charlie and his long-term partner had got engaged (what finally convinced her to take the plunge with this man I was never quite sure; it certainly can't have been his sense of humour). Spotting Rana on the ward not long after, I asked her how she was feeling about the (presumably devastating) news of her unrequited love's engagement.

"Oh, I don't really care," Rana replied, in a surprisingly off-handed tone. "To be honest, I don't even fancy Charlie anymore. Have you seen him recently? He's got this massive spot on his forehead that completely puts you off even looking at him. Honestly, it's so big it's practically an abscess."

"I don't know, Rana," I replied, tongue very much firmly in cheek, "it sounds like you've still got a bit of a fixation on Charlie. I mean, you're clearly *abscessed* with him."

You know, it's at moments like this that I suddenly find myself wondering what convinced my wife to marry me. Sadly, I'm reasonably certain that my penchant for puns hasn't got much better over the years.

ST2 (GERIATRICS): IF I HAD TO DO THE SAME AGAIN...

There is a subtle yet unmistakeable expression you are bound to see adorn the face of most doctors at some point, if you spend enough time with them. If I had to describe it, I would call it a look of repressed exasperation, or simply 'the look'. It's an expression that's typically provoked by a patient telling us something either painfully unfunny, highly questionable, or downright incredulous. Our training and sense of professional decorum do thankfully kick in, but often not *quite* enough to fully suppress the inevitable look of disbelief, shock or frustration that follows the patient's comment. We are human, after all.

At times, patients will genuinely make you laugh, often because they've said something (typically at an unexpected moment) that genuinely throws you. Sometimes, patients will do this deliberately in order to ease the tension of an uncomfortable situation. One of my favourite examples of this was a young man who, shortly after I had performed a rectal examination on him, said, "Sheesh, at least buy me dinner first next time."

Sometimes, the patient is not trying to be funny at all. I'll certainly never forget the lady in her eighties whom I looked after on the Geriatrics ward, who had delusional disorder, and was absolutely convinced her daughter was in some way plotting against her. "Do you know, doctor, my daughter came to visit me earlier," she told me one afternoon. "While she was here, I was determined to scrutinise her every facial expression, hoping to expose her lies. But no matter how hard I tried, I simply couldn't read her face. Then again, ever since she's been on those steroid tablets for her joints, she's got so fat that *no one* can read her face." To laugh in that moment would surely have been the height of unprofessionalism, and thankfully I didn't. My God, it wasn't easy though.

When patients are intentionally trying to be funny, the jokes certainly don't always land. The longer you do this job, the more you inevitably start hearing some of the same tired old clangers – and in those moments, you just don't have the heart to tell your patient (as they marvel at their own spontaneous 'hilarity') that you've heard said line at least a hundred times before. Cliché it may be, but if I had a pound coin for every time a patient has replied to the question, 'Do you have any allergies?' with the answer 'doctors', 'hospitals', or 'just the wife' I'd be a multi-millionaire. You still try to force a polite laugh (or at least a smile), but 'the look' often can't help but come through as well. And the more senior you become, the more and more that same look involuntarily gets wheeled out.

The undisputed king of 'the look' was my Geriatrics consultant, Dr Fernando. An affable, well-spoken African man in his fifties, Dr Fernando was the type of kind, supportive boss I had long pined for during some of my earlier surgical rotations as an FY1 and FY2 (with the possible exception of Mr Franks, my T&O consultant). Originally born in Nigeria, I think it's fair to say Dr Fernando and I didn't look remotely alike (and with me being Arabic, why would we?). However, that still didn't stop one of the Geriatrics' nurses from once telling me I looked like I was "his illegitimate lovechild." Clearly, despite changing jobs, hospitals and geographical regions, nothing had really changed since the moment I'd been asked, straight-faced, by a nurse just over two years earlier (while working in Cardiology) whether I was black. Apparently, the 'evidence' was mounting...

But again, I digress.

The first time I saw Dr Fernando bust out 'the look' was during a ward round early into my four-month rotation under his supervision. We were reviewing an elderly gentleman with Alzheimer's disease, who had three weeks earlier fallen on the ward and broken his hip, necessitating emergency surgery. However, due to his severe dementia, the patient very soon forgot all about the fall, the fracture, and even the fact he had had surgery.

"Hello, sir," Dr Fernando said as he kneeled down beside the patient. "How's your hip doing today?"

"What?" came the confused reply.

"How's *your hip*?" Dr Fernando said again, a little louder.

"My what?" the patient replied, still utterly lost.

"Your *hip*, sir. I want to know how your *hip* is."

"Hip?" the patient said, bemused. After considering Dr Fernando's question for a moment, a wry smile broke out across the patient's face. "Hip hip hooray!"

Now, I thought this was pretty funny (and still do). Dr Fernando, however, had clearly heard this joke before – and seemingly not just the once. Cue 'the look'.

However, the most memorable, and also unexpected, appearance of 'the look' came about during a conversation Dr Fernando had with Derek, the son of an elderly gentleman under our care, who sadly had terminal metastatic cancer. One of the sad realities of working in Geriatrics is that you end up having difficult conversations with patients and their relatives on a fairly frequent basis, ones in which, invariably, you tell them everything they most likely don't want to hear.

Derek lived some distance away from the hospital, and the day we encountered him on the ward was his first time visiting his father as an inpatient, as well as his first time meeting his father's consultant, Dr Fernando. We ushered Derek into a quiet side room, sat him down, and closed the door. With his usual tact and gentle manner, Dr Fernando explained to Derek that, sadly, there were no further active treatments we were able to offer his father and, therefore, our main priority moving forwards was just to keep him comfortable. The tone of the meeting was understandably sombre. Derek remained mostly silent throughout, presumably trying to make sense in his head of everything he was being told.

As the meeting ended, Derek stood up, shook Dr Fernando's hand, and headed for the door. "I really appreciate your time today, doctor," Derek said as he turned back to Dr Fernando. "As you know, I live quite a way away, and so don't know how often I'll physically be able to come down here. If I do have any further questions, would it be okay if I gave you a ring?"

"Of course," Dr Fernando affirmed. "You can reach me via my secretary if you call the hospital switchboard number."

"Thank you, doctor. I'm really sorry to ask, but I actually didn't quite catch your name at the very beginning..."

"Not to worry," the consultant replied. "It's Dr Fernando."

With those three words, Derek's entire demeanour changed in an instant. As a mischievous smile broke out across his face, Derek said, "Oh, well I'll have no problem remembering that!"

And with that, as Derek turned the door handle and exited the side room, he suddenly adopted an almost spring in his step, and launched into a tone-deaf rendition of the chorus to *Fernando* by ABBA.

Utilising every fibre of my being not to laugh, I couldn't help but turn to look at Dr Fernando, as Derek's warbling singing trailed off into the distance. Yes, 'the look' was very much in full force once more. And if I had to translate the thinly concealed expression of chagrin on Dr Fernando's face, it surely read: "For fuck's sake – not *again*."

ST3 (PAEDIATRICS): LAST ARAB STANDING (AKA BLEACH BLONDE)

And so it was that three years and eight months, three hospitals and ten job posts after finishing medical school, I began what was to be my final ever hospital attachment: Paediatrics. Although I ultimately did very much enjoy the rotation (mainly as I love working with kids), I also couldn't help but look to the future. After this post was over, I'd be doing a straight sixteen-month stretch in General Practice before – hopefully – having my training wheels well and truly removed for good, and being sent out into the big wide world as a bona fide GP. No more twelve-hour hospital on calls; no more night shifts; and no more eccentric hospital colleagues to have to put up with on a daily basis. I couldn't wait. But fate, it seemed, wasn't about to let me off that easily.

During my four months in Paediatrics, it's not an understatement to say I was the most consistently ill I had ever been, before or since (with the possible exception of when my son first went to nursery...). Over the course of those seventeen weeks, in quick succession I suffered from: glandular fever (a viral illness which left me with a golf ball-sized lump in my neck that persisted for several weeks); episcleritis (an inflammatory condition that affects the outer layer of the eye);

bacterial tonsillitis (a throat infection that floored me to the extent that it forced me to call in sick for two successive night shifts, something I had previously never even *contemplated* doing, much less actually done); hand, foot & mouth (a viral illness that causes mouth ulcers, plus blister formation over the hands and feet); and finally, impetigo (a highly contagious skin infection). I knew why this had happened, of course; neither I nor my immune system were used to dealing with so many ill children, and so it was perhaps inevitable I would pick up a few of the conditions I was treating. However, I also couldn't help but feel at times that this was fate's way of punishing me for daring to leave hospital medicine behind, deciding to try to finish me off before I could finish the rotation. As a result, my four months in Paediatrics ended up being a much tougher physical slog than I had anticipated. By the end, I didn't so much cross the finish line as collapse in a feeble heap just beyond it.

My final hospital clinical supervisor was a consultant called Dr Radisson. A well-to-do, bespectacled woman in her fifties with greying blonde hair, Dr Radisson was posh with a capital P, and whenever you heard her genteel voice you couldn't help but be reminded of Hyacinth Bucket from British sitcom classic *Keeping Up Appearances*.

Dr Radisson was also a devout Christian, and would always be seen sporting her trademark silver cross around her neck. When we did weekend on calls together, she would even excuse herself for two hours on a Sunday (leaving behind me and a registrar) so that she could attend the morning service at her local church. Yes, Dr Radisson was most definitely old school; indeed, I soon learned she was perhaps a little *too* old school.

During one particular on call shift, about a month into my rotation, I was preparing to review a two-year-old child (Thomas) on the Paediatric Admissions Unit, who had been brought in with a fever and a widespread rash. Looking through his notes, I spotted a clinic letter dated a few months earlier which had been signed by Dr Radisson. It transpired that Thomas had been seen in Dr Radisson's outpatient clinic after having been referred by his GP with severe eczema, and Dermatology (the branch of medicine dealing with the skin) happened to be one of Dr Radisson's specialist interests. Scanning through the letter, I was struck and, moreover, alarmed by one particular sentence that appeared in the penultimate paragraph: *I have also advised mother that, when she is bathing Thomas, she should apply half a cupful of bleach to the bath water.*

Bleach?! Was this for real? I was, to put it mildly, stunned. Had this just been an *extremely* unfortunate typo? Or, worse still, was this a genuine piece of medical advice that a Paediatrics consultant had given on how to treat a two-year-old's eczema?

As I came across more and more of Dr Raddison's clinic letters, it very quickly became clear that what I had read in that initial document was no typo; Dr Raddison, it seemed, was routinely advising diluting bleach in bath water as a treatment for children with eczema. I couldn't believe it.

A quick search of Dermatology literature online did, fortunately, allay my fears somewhat. As bewildering and unlikely as it sounds, diluted bleach is indeed, in some circles, used as a treatment for severe cases of eczema, as it kills harmful bacteria that live on the skin's surface (in a similar vein to the chlorine in swimming pools). However, most clinicians nowadays regard this treatment as, to put it charitably, outdated, and so no longer recommend it to patients; it's certainly not something I've ever advised as a GP – if I did, it's not entirely farfetched to think I might then end up being reported to the General Medical Council (GMC).

As part of my GP training scheme, I was fortunate to be able to attend outpatient clinics in a variety of medical disciplines, as a means of further broadening my knowledge and experience. One of these disciplines – the clinics for which almost coincided with my time in Paediatrics – just happened to be Dermatology. During one such clinic, in a quiet moment between patients, I couldn't help but ask the consultant I was sat in with that day, Dr Hill, as to his thoughts on the use of diluted bleach in the management of children with eczema. What I was expecting was a dispassionate, reasoned explanation as to the clinical justification behind the use of this treatment. To my surprise, what I got instead was an expression of abject horror. His mouth slightly agape, Dr Hill's simple response was a stunned, "*Shit...*"

I remember my very last shift in hospital medicine very well. It was, as it happened, a night shift (the third of three consecutive nights I had done), and frustratingly, I was ill – again. Given just how many times I had been unwell over the preceding four months though, I was hardly surprised.

On this occasion, I had impetigo (though I didn't know that at first). I had felt a bit rough during the preceding night shift, but was determined to come in for this final one. After all, this was going to be my last ever hospital shift. Also, after feeling I had let my colleagues down a few months earlier when I was forced to call in sick for two night shifts because of tonsillitis, I wasn't about to do the same again if I could at all avoid it, no matter how ill I may have felt.

I can't say that it was the easiest or most pleasant twelve-hour shift I'd ever done but, buoyed by a strong sense of resolve and determination, I just about got through it. What didn't help matters was that shortly after the shift began, I noticed I had come out in a red, weepy rash over my face, which only became more extensive and nastier-looking as the night went on. *Damn*, I thought, *the hospital really is determined to finish me off*.

Fortunately though, I won out in the end.

As the morning handover meeting concluded, and I left the ward office for what would be the final time, I happened to catch sight of myself in a nearby mirror. It was, to be frank, not a pretty sight. In a way though, it was almost symbolic: it looked for all the world like I'd been visibly scarred – not just by the impetigo, and the physical toll the rotation had taken on me, but by the entire punishing three-plus years in hospital medicine. In short, I looked rough – and, like an idiot, I hadn't even brought my diluted bleach concealer with me to work that day.

And, with that, it was over. Aside from a few low-key goodbyes from the registrar and consultant I had been on call with overnight, no one would've guessed this was anything other than the end of a perfectly normal night shift. And, in some ways, it was. Yet for me, despite the lack of any fanfare (or, indeed, almost any sense of occasion) there most definitely was something different about that morning – and not just the unfortunate rash on my face. In spite of the fact I still had sixteen months left of my training, that day truly felt like the culmination of a very long, frequently difficult, often frustrating, but ultimately defining chapter in my life.

Despite all the dramas of the preceding few years (or, perhaps, because of them) I really felt like I had accomplished something, and taken a massive step forward in my journey towards becoming a GP. But that, of course, meant having to say goodbye to hospital medicine for good.

As I grabbed my belongings and finally left the ward, I tried to take it all in: the hubbub of morning handover between the nursing staff; the familiar beeping of monitors in the near distance; the sound of children eating their breakfast; and the fresh sunlight streaming in through the windows, bathing the ward in its early April light. Life on the wards would of course go on, as it always had – but for me, it was over.

As the enormity of that moment washed over me, I suddenly found myself briefly resembling the aforementioned Dermatologist, Dr Hill – mouth slightly agape, mostly lost for words, and thinking silently to myself:

Shit...

Though I have always considered it somewhat pretentious when writers choose to conclude their work with a quote, I must confess I can think of no better way to finish this book than with the following quote by author Ursula K. Le Guin. In many ways, it encapsulates a time in my life that, though often testing and trying, remains a vital part of my medical journey, left an indelible mark, and helped mould my character in more ways than I could have ever foreseen on that very first Black Wednesday, all those years ago: 'It is good to have an end to journey towards; but it is the journey that matters, in the end'.

AFTERWORD

In writing this book and reflecting on my experiences in hospital medicine (some of which were more than a decade ago now), it struck me just how eclectic a group of individuals I had worked alongside over the course of my four or so years as a hospital doctor. Watching those doctors deal with specific situations – from fawning over private patients on a florally named hospital suite, to squirting water in the face of unsuspecting individuals with psychological issues – was frequently revealing, surprising, and sometimes just downright horrifying.

In many ways, how as doctors we deal with death often very much speaks to our character, and to the types of people we are. As a junior doctor in hospitals, one of the grim but necessary duties is to officially certify the death of patients who have passed away. And, morbid though it may sound, reading the various ways in which different doctors would choose to document their verification of death in the medical notes was always fascinating to me.

Some doctors would be very clinical, and almost overly formal in their approach: *I do therefore hereby declare that Mr Clarke has expired*, wrote one.

Other doctors (often, I suspected, the ones who were quite religious) would become almost spiritual in their documentation: *I can confirm that Mr Patel has sadly died. May his eternal soul rest in heavenly peace.*

And then there were some who were blunt (often brutally so) and to the point: *Asked by the nurses to confirm that Mr Cox has died. [List of patient observations.] Conclusion: Mr Cox is dead.*

These are but three examples of just how much variety exists amongst healthcare professionals. Inevitably, that sometimes means that different personalities are almost certainly bound to clash – my repeated run-ins with The Dragon Lady perhaps exemplifies that philosophy better than anything.

But as the years pass, I'm realising more and more just how important those distinct voices that make up the tapestry of our NHS are, principally because of the equally varied voices and personality types we see amongst patients. Perhaps, in the end, it all balances out. After all, as I myself found during my time in O&G, there are people who will respect, and even *like* a dragon, whether that appreciation is something I can personally ever understand or not. Ultimately, such things are always going to be subjective – and for me, that's perhaps been the most important lesson of all.

I do appreciate that many of the experiences recounted within this book may come across as overly negative. Whilst they are all entirely true, it must be said that they are also not wholly representative of my complete junior doctor experience. Over the course of my time working in hospital medicine, I also came across all manner of hard-working, empathetic, professional and inspiring individuals. Had I not, I would undoubtedly have become disillusioned with the profession long before I crossed the finish line to qualify as a

GP. The simple (yet hopefully not overly cynical) truth is that any stories I have about *those* people are just not as captivating – as George Bernard Shaw once remarked, 'No conflict, no drama'. But I don't want to appear in any way disingenuous; such positive forces for good absolutely do exist within our NHS, and I've been fortunate and proud to work alongside more than just a fair share. And with any luck, I shall continue to do so for many years to come.

That being said, there's bound to be some more quacks along the way, too...